LIVINGOOD DAILY

YOUR 21-DAY GUIDE TO EXPERIENCE REAL HEALTH + WORKBOOK

DR. LIVINGOOD

Livingood Daily
Your 21-Day Guide to Experience Real Health + Workbook
ISBN-13: 978-1975838997
By Dr. Livingood

Revision 2.0 1st Printing, July 2020
Printed in the United States of America

Dedication

To dad, for bringing me into this world and helping me find out why. May this book and its message change millions of lives in your honor.

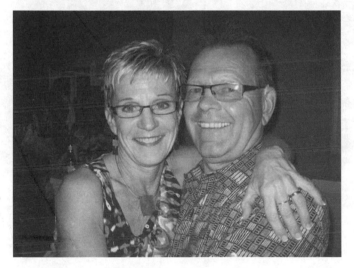

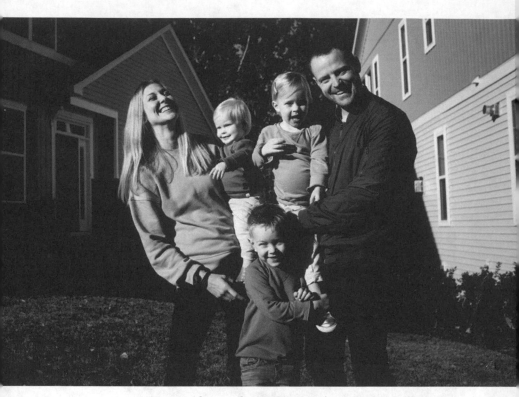

*If you focus on sickness and disease,
you get sickness and disease.
If you focus on health and the activities
of building health, you get health.*

CONTENTS

CHAPTER 1 THE $15,000,000 CHECK 1

2 EXPERIENCE REAL HEALTH 11

3 THE LIVINGOOD DAILY FORMULA 20

4 REMOVE THE INTERFERENCE 36

5 FIX YOUR FOCUS 46

6 FIX YOUR FOOD 62

7 FIX YOUR FITNESS 84

8 FIX YOUR FRAME 92

9 FIX YOUR FILTERS 105

10 1% PROGRESS TO LIVINGOOD DAILY 118

CITATIONS 137

SUPPLEMENT GUIDE 142

CHALLENGE WORKBOOK 150

1

If you don't take care of your body, where will you live?

CHAPTER ONE
THE $15,000,000 CHECK

Is there something you know you should be doing for your health right now and are simply not doing it? Procrastination is the THIEF of health. Most people are working their whole life to gain wealth in order to retire, but they're expending their health doing it. Then, they retire and have to spend all of their wealth trying to regain their health.

What good is the paycheck, the stress, all the busyness, the nice things, or the career, if you don't have your health during, or after it?

After leading hundreds of thousands of people to live good daily, I have found a clear answer to what many really want at the end of the day. If you are reading this book, then I know you are an action taker that wants more in life.

This book is a simple, quick read to do one thing: Light a

fire under you to act NOW. To get you from "I SHOULD eat better with more movement,", and be consistent with I MUST. If you need a novel, this isn't your book. You don't need more information. You need knowledge. People perish for lack of knowledge. Knowledge is the application of information. DO. Do not just read. Do not just take the information. DO. Alternatively—Do! Don't just read. Don't just take in information. Do! If I can get you to realize the urgency of DOING the plan this book will give you, then I have done my job as a doctor, which means teacher.

If you want to add life to your years not just years to your life, if you want life and health now while you work, if you want life once you retire—the beach, grandkids, adventure, energy, if you want to dictate life on your terms instead of sickness calling the shots—this is your guide.

This is your guide if you are sick and tired of being sick and tired, and you are ready for your comeback. Or, like me, if you have seen the loss of health and devastation of disease destroy a loved one's life and are committed to that not being you.

What is the biggest asset that you have? What is the most important thing that you own? What is the biggest gift you have been given? It's you. It's you. It's you. You are the biggest asset that you have. You are no good to your job, to your family, or to your purpose if you're sick or dead. The book you hold is intended to help you to experience real health;—not sickness, disease, and early death—and to live life to the fullest, avoid stress, find your purpose, and reach your full potential. You cannot accomplish what you've been put here to do if you do not have your health.

Most of us have everything that we need to be successful, to be happy, and to be healthy. All the potential and power is within us—we're just messing it up. We're interfering with our own greatness. This book is your guide so that you can remove the interference in your health. A healthier you leads you to live the life and be the person you were created to be. This book aims to inspire you to take action and make deposits in the biggest investment you can possibly make an investment in... YOU!

Imagine a $15,000,000 blank check in my hand. I'm filling out the check with your name. In an instant, you can deposit millions into your bank account. You are going to pay off your debt. You can pick what car you want. What would you pick? I'd go for the 1967 Ford Mustang. Where would your new house be? Who would you buy lavish gifts for? What good would you do for people? Imagine the possibilities and doors that 15 million dollars will provide!

Here's the catch. In return for that $15,000,000... I get your arms and legs. They will be removed from your body. Do you take the deal?

OF COURSE YOU DON'T! I already know your answer. What good are the car, the house, and the trips if you can't walk or move! That means your arms and legs are worth at least $15 million! Would you trade your heart? Your eyes? Your tongue? NO!

Right now, you are sitting, literally, on millions! The vehicle called your body is more valuable than all the things and money in this world! How are you treating it?

If you had a $100,000 car how would you treat it? How do you treat your $10,000 car? Do you maintain it? Change the oil?

Wash it? Fuel it with the right fuel? Clean it? Then, why are you abusing the only vehicle you get for this journey called life? Most take better care of their cars than their own vehicle, their body! There are no trade-ins, no leasing, and no rentals; you get one vehicle for the whole ride, and it's up to you how long the ride lasts. I learned this the hard way.

Health is your biggest asset.

It was the fall of 2007. I remember exactly where I was on that day—I was getting my doctorate. I was in class, and I stepped out into the hallway. I remember the pattern on the carpet— it was made up of different-colored squares. My phone was ringing, and I answered to hear someone bawling on the other end.

"Mom, what's wrong?" I asked.

She said, "Your dad's heart just shut down; he is being airlifted to Mayo Clinic."

Now, this is a phone call I would never wish on anyone. The shock of these scenarios is some of the worst we face on this earth. As shocking as that would be, regardless of whom it was, it was especially shocking because it was my dad. My father had no symptoms, was on no medications, had no health ailments that we knew of, and had passed 30 plus years of physicals working for UPS. How could he possibly be unhealthy?

We spent the next couple of weeks fighting to get to the bottom of my dad's problem. He had an electrical shortage leading to his heart, but we couldn't figure out what was causing it. Over the next few weeks, I learned first-hand the life lesson that the biggest asset we have is our health—not just our own health, but the health of everyone that we love. When you lose your health, or a loved one loses their health, what can you do tomorrow? Nothing. You can't work, you can't have fun, and you can't live your purpose. Health is the physical foundation of it all.

Over the next two years, I saw my dad go through something that I would like to prevent every human being from going through, and that is... the American healthcare system! In two years, my dad ended up on 15-plus different medications. They put him on so much Prednisone that it ate the cartilage out of his knees and nose and swelled his face like a balloon. They sawed up through his chest and performed open-heart surgery, installing a fake valve.

My dad lost his hearing on January 5th, never to hear his grandbabies' voices again, never to hear his wife's real voice again, and never to enjoy the sound of the 70's rock music that he loved. His hearing was gone because of all the inflammation in his body.

Can you hear right now? Have you ever thought about how miraculous that is? Do you realize how much of a gift it is to be able to wake up every day and hear, see, and taste? There are people in this world who can't, and we take it for granted.

To try to hear our voices again, doctors installed metal plates and cochlear implants as fake ears into dad's head. By the time dad was 53, he was partly bionic and bedridden for multiple days a week. He couldn't work and provide for his family; in fact, he never worked again. Blow after blow, this piled up and cost my family well over $200,000 in medical procedures. I remember the day my mom received a bill in the mail for one injection my dad had received. The invoice read $20,000 for one injection! Needless to say, that was a bad day for our family and my dad was still sicker than ever.

The worst part of losing your health?
Losing your potential and your purpose!

My dad's condition ripped him away from his purpose of providing for his family, going fishing with his two boys, going biking with my mom, enjoying holidays, etc. He was ripped away from all the things that mattered. He couldn't even go to church! My dad lost his biggest asset; therefore, he lost everything.

What is the biggest asset that you have been given? It's you! If you don't have your health, you can't fulfill the purpose that you're here to do.

My father wasn't missing any parts, he didn't need fake parts, he didn't need another drug—he needed healing! The wounds were self-inflicted, as healthy as my dad thought he was. We started to realize he was causing it by the subtle things you and I do every day that interfere with our health.

Through the test of my dad losing his health, I realized being a doctor wasn't just a job for me, but it was a purpose, a calling. The process of getting my dad well is what millions of people were, and are, praying for all over the world. Within a ten-mile radius around you right now, thousands of people are suffering, prayer lists are getting longer, and more disease exists now than ever before in America. Health care, if you can call it that, is a mess. I realized God could use my dad's health loss as a purpose for my life to not only save him but many others—I just had to get the potential in me.

The information in this book and in the coming chapters is the road that led me to find answers for my dad to not only save his life but to go on and save hundreds of thousands of other lives. A decade or two ago, if my dad could have picked up the book that you're holding right now, it could have changed everything for my family.

All things work together for good, and I believe that my dad suffered so thousands can get help! The biggest test of my life has now turned into my biggest testimony to help you and your family experience real health.

No one will take better care of you...
than you!

Results matter. To encourage you, I filled this book with real people taking massive action and changing their lives. Why? To make this a picture book? No, to show you that YOU CAN. The biggest mistake people make is that they never start. They think they've tried it all or don't need to. If you had tried it all, you'd be fixed by now.

I believe we have complicated and confused the world with nutrition and diets. This book will put the confusion to death. Health isn't complicated if you don't let it be. Some of you are addicted to making matters complicated and controversial. If we'd just spend more time following the laws of what a human needs to thrive, we'd build a lot more health.

Can it really be simple? Yes. Notice I didn't say easy. Change is not easy, but it's worth it. I will give you all you need, regardless of what you are up against, to change your life now. I will show you the faces of people that have overcome nearly any condition you can think of to show that YOU can do it too.

You have to make a decision and take massive action with it. You can read this book in two hours, but apply its teachings for 20 years. You don't need 400 pages of HOW. You need one big WHY. Today is your turning point. Today is your moment. You MUST change. You will never be the same again. This one little book can be the spark for YOU to change it all. If you have no other resource than that mentality, then you can do this.

To let you know what's possible on your journey, read what happened in 4 weeks in a small church in Angier, NC, with this book.

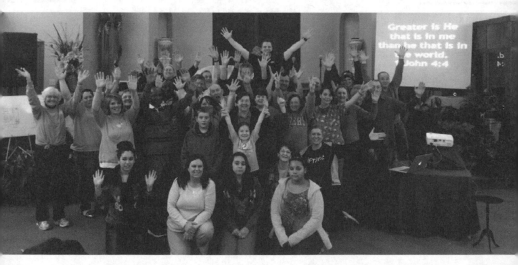

- In four weeks of applying Livingood Daily, this group of 35 people lost over 500 pounds!
- One lady has lost 115 pounds in 11 months!

- One pastor came off several heart medications for an incurable condition. Both pastors lost over 30 pounds each.
- A man who was unable to work due to a stroke is now off a few medications, strong, and back to work.
- A child with Asperger Syndrome is now highly functional in a normal school, baffling the school nurse.
- Several people came off blood pressure medications.
- A little boy with a four-year infection and compromised immune system was healed in four weeks.
- A child came off an asthma inhaler.
- A single mom no longer suffers from back pain.
- Another single mom has a decreased thyroid issue, more energy, better digestion, and no more back pain.
- A child avoided having scoliosis surgery.
- A woman's digestive problems are gone, and her husband's neck pain is, too.
- A grandfather who suffered a stroke came off his blood pressure medication and can now hold his grandbaby again.
- Dozens of others have continued to receive health, never getting sick in the first place.

What I love about this church is that they don't have a lot of resources, gyms, or health food stores, but they excelled and did it anyway! They made a decision: "We are going to change." They did it together, and so will we. By the end of this book, not only will I give you the mentality and tools, but I will show you how to get connected with thousands of others along this exact journey with you.

First, you need the right knowledge.
People perish without it.

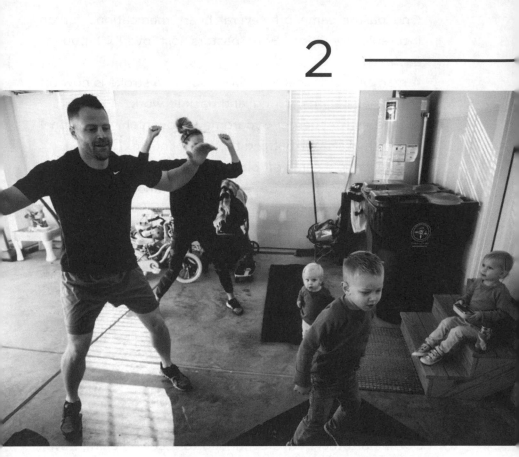

"There really is no system of health care in this country now. It's like going to the garage to try to fix your car, and when you get to the garage you realize you don't have a car. You can't fix something that doesn't exist."

- Dr. Denis Cortese, Mayo Clinic's Chief Executive and President

CHAPTER TWO
EXPERIENCE REAL HEALTH

How are we doing when it comes to being healthy in the USA? When you look at the state of health care in America right now, it's staggering how sick we've become. This chapter is meant to do one thing: WAKE YOU UP so that you stop thinking you SHOULD get health and finally decide you MUST get healthy. There is no choice. No turning back to old ways. The time is now, or you will end up a statistic. Don't think it will be you? Here are the facts.

Ask 100 people right now, "Do you plan on getting a major disease (heart disease, cancer, etc.) in your lifetime?" Most, if not all, of them, will say, "No, not me!" Yet, current statistics show that seven out of 10 Americans die of chronic disease.[1] Five out of six Americans (83%) get heart disease or cancer in their lifetime![2, 3] How do you explain this?

People think they are healthier than they actually are.

No one thinks they'll get a disease, so they just ignore doing the things necessary to maintain health.

Medicine, our current healthcare system, was created to save a life in crisis (heart attack, car accident, etc.). Thank God for that, but it is NOT designed to get someone healthy; you cannot give a drug to a person and expect them to get healthier. Most Americans wait until they are sick and then rely on a drug or surgery to try to get them healthy. The consequences of this have been devastating.

If you had a pond full of sick fish, how would you fix it?

Would you pour drugs into the pond?
Would you take the fish out and perform micro fish surgery?
Would you dissect the fish and analyze their genetics?
No.
You'd clean up the water! Medicine is not cleaning up the water; in fact, it is just making it more toxic.

America has the worst modernized healthcare system on the planet. Johns Hopkins University rated the top 37 industrialized nations, and America was dead last in overall health care—yet we're spending more than any other country.[4, 5] Almost 34% of Americans are considered obese, 35% of whom are children aged five to 17. We have more violence and injuries, more sexually-transmitted diseases, and more obesity. We also have

13

more chronic lung disease, more heart disease, and more diabetes than almost anywhere else on the planet.[5]

Last year, Americans spent $2.6 trillion in health care; that's almost 18% of our gross domestic product. We spend nearly $9,000 per year, per person on health care. When you look at other countries like Germany, France, Italy, or Norway, they're spending nearly half as much as we are; yet when you look at our overall health, we are doing worse than them.[5]

We have more death from disease and injury per 100,000 people than those countries.[5] Our first-day death rate is 69th in the world, and our infant mortality rate (the percentage of babies who die within the first year) is 26th out of industrialized countries.[6, 7] Infant mortality is widely considered a key indicator of the health of a country, and we're near the bottom of the industrialized world. Our life expectancy is 53rd in the world right now: you could live in 52 other countries and live longer than you do here.[8]

Our healthcare system does not exist. We've turned to man to create a healthcare system, but it's not a healthcare system. When do you go see a doctor in America? When you're already sick. If you pass a physical, what do doctors do to you? NOTHING! See you next year. That means you have to be sick in order to enter the system--that's not a healthcare system; that's a sick-care system.

"There really is no system of health care in this country now."
- Denis Cortese, President of Mayo Clinic, 2006

Dr. Denis Cortese, Mayo Clinic's chief executive and president, was asked, "How would you fix our broken health care system?" He said, "There really is no system of health care in this country now." He referred to it as "going to the garage to try to fix your car, but when you get to the garage, you realize you don't have a car. You can't fix something that doesn't exist."

In 2006, when my father was sick, Dr. Cortese was the man running the hospital where my dad was being treated. Our family paid thousands of dollars to them. We put our faith in them to restore my father's health; but, the leader of the facility, at the same time, was saying health care didn't exist there.

Our system is broken. $750 billion dollars are spent annually just on unnecessary services, delivery of care, administrative costs, and fraud.[9] We're throwing money out the window and we're not getting any results in return.

The percentage of doctors who are paid based on the quality of care they deliver is 30% in the United States; that means there's only incentive to give quality care for 30% of the procedures done. In places like the U.K., it's 95%. Our spending is through the roof, but our results are not there.[9]

In 2013, The American Health Organization rated America overall worst in efficiency, cost, quality, and results. Seventy percent of Americans are on a prescription drug plan, which includes twenty-five percent of all children.[10, 11] We take 25 million pills per hour in America.

The British Medical Journal stated in 1991 that only about 15% of medical interventions are supported by solid, scientific evidence.[12] 20% of Americans experience some form of malpractice in their lifetime; 18% of hospital patients suffer an injury during the course of their care; one in seven Medicare patients suffer injuries during their hospital stay. Up to 40 wrong-site, wrong-side, wrong-patient, or wrong-procedure surgeries happen weekly in the United States; adverse events during medical care contribute to 180,000 deaths per year; nine times more people will die annually from adverse medical events than will die from firearms.[9]

It is evident that the American medical system is in the top three leading causes of death and injury in the United States, if not the first.[13] The Book and Documentary *Death By Medicine* sheds light on the total number of deaths being created by our health care system by adding together mistakes in hospitals, mistakes with surgeries, medical errors, infections in hospitals, malnutrition in hospitals, and drug-reaction deaths; and the total is more than 800,000 deaths per year in America! This death rate is more than heart disease and more than cancer.

Our system is not only not working and failing us miserably, but it has now become the number-one cause of harm. I do not see a bigger problem facing Americans today than our healthcare crisis; it's bankrupting our country, it's taking away our health, it's destroying our marriages, and it's taking people away from their potential.

It's costing us--it's costing us incredibly. The number one cause of bankruptcy in the United States today is medical bills. Medical bills account for 62% of bankruptcies: 78% of those people had health insurance but went bankrupt anyway. 14 Man's solution–insurance and medicine–is not working.

Starbucks and General Motors spend more on health care than they do on making coffee and steel for cars.[15, 16] The best financial seminar we could put on for anyone in America is a health seminar to get to the cause of issues, correct the problems, and experience real health.

In 2009, the Journal of American Medical Association stated that data remains imprecise that the benefits U.S. healthcare currently delivers do not outweigh the aggregate health harm it implies.[17]

One of our top medical journals states that the benefit of our healthcare system does not outweigh the harm of our health care system! When something causes more harm than good, we have to change.

"There is a way that seems right to a man, but its end is the way of death."
– Proverbs 14:12

There's a way that may seem right to get someone healthy, but it leads to death. There's a way that seems right to insure people and give them more benefits, but in the end, it leads to death. Although a drug or a surgery may save a life in a crisis, the side effects and lack of fixing the cause of the problem leads to death. If a solution doesn't build health, then it shouldn't belong in a healthcare system. We MUST distinguish between healthcare and crisis/sick care.

I experience this in my own backyard. I live in the state of North Carolina, in what is referred to as the Research Triangle. It is one of the country's epicenters for advancement in "health" care, and some of the nation's top doctors and researchers work here. The funny thing is that North Carolina is by no means the healthiest place in the country; in fact, we are sicker than most. North Carolina is rated as the 37th state in the country in overall health. We have more medical care, immunizations, and doctors than nearly any place in the world, yet we rank 37th.[18] Additionally, people in our churches are some of the sickest.

I believe churches should be the healthiest places on the planet, but that is not the case. A recent study that compared self-reported chronic diseases in parishioners who go to churches in North Carolina found that there was a 41% obesity rate, a 36% high blood pressure rate, a 34% arthritis rate, a 14% asthma rate, and a 13% diabetes rate. When you compare the people in the church to people outside the church, people in the church had 10% more obesity, 4% more blood pressure, 2.5% more arthritis, 4.1% more asthma, and 3.3% more diabetes.[19]

The point isn't to stop attending church; the point is that we MUST start delivering real health to churches, businesses, schools, and the general population, or else these results will only get worse.

I've done this long enough to know that I have to spend at least 50% of my effort just waking you up, motivating you, inspiring you, and empowering you to believe that you MUST take care of your health. The "how" will be easy if the "why" is right.

At the end of the day, your health is whose responsibility? It's your own. If you leave it to some insurance company, workplace, doctor, or man to take care of, well...just reflect on those statistics and consider the likely outcome.

"No one is coming for you!"

Building health is up to you. Big pharma and big food want you sick and addicted. They profit off it. You want health? Go get it. You MUST.

You have a choice when it comes to your health. You can take this information, apply, and do something different. However, if you ignore it and take the same approach as everyone else around you, then what will you end up with? The same results as everybody else. All these stats and studies show that it would mean sickness, disease, bankruptcy, and early death.

You MUST take charge of your health. I encourage you to see the trouble in front of you and what lies ahead. Don't just hide from it, but take action to avoid it. Ignoring your health and not changing your ways leads to further problems and you're ultimately suffering the consequences. Empower yourself with the tools that follow to change your life, and take the path to Livingood Daily.

REVERSED CANCER AND HAS LOST WEIGHT!

IS 5 YEARS CANCER FREE AND OFFICIALLY CANCER FREE!

YEARS OF DIABETES AND MEDS GONE IN A FEW WEEKS!

3

*Greater is He that is in you than
he that is in the world.*
- 1 John 4:4

*"What lies behind you and what lies in front of you
pales in comparison to what lies inside of you."*
- Ralph Waldo Emerson

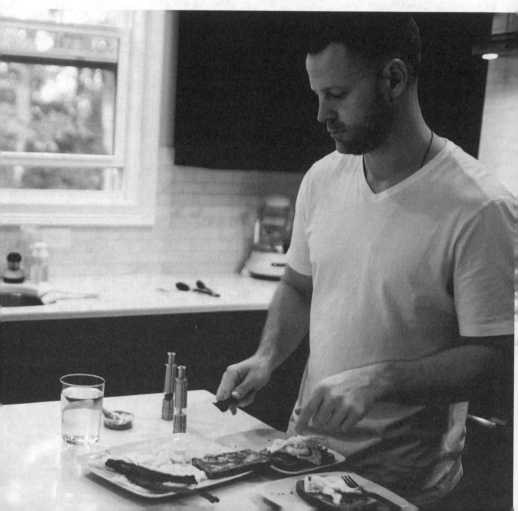

CHAPTER THREE

THE LIVINGOOD DAILY FORMULA

There's a power inside of you!

The difference between you and a dead person is POWER; it runs through you and heals you. If that power can work, you can; without that power, you have no potential. I believe the reason people don't experience real health is that they don't truly understand that power or know what health is in the first place. But first, where are you trying to go?

We must begin with the end in mind. You have to know where you are going. If you want to go to Florida and you drive West, there is no chance you will get there. You can drive as fast as you want but you are simply going in the wrong direction. If you want to get to another level of health, break through and get the pounds off, get back to the shape you used to be in, get a solid exercise regimen, correct the cause of the ailments that you have, and experience less stress, get off medications, and live up to your full potential, then you've got to start with that end in mind. In your workbook, there is room every day to write down what you want to see happen in the next 30 days and over the next 30 years. Write it down. Mark an "X" on your map so you know where you are going.

Health is not a program!

There are no shortcuts to your destination. If you want to climb Mount Everest, you need to develop strength, endurance, and knowledge along the way to survive the climb. There are no helicopter "program" rides to the top. You have to condition yourself to have a healthy climb. Health is a climb. To get into "peak" health takes work. It's why most people stay on the flat ground and resort to drugs and quick fixes. Put to death dieting, programs, and pills, because all they are doing is weakening your true strength for the journey.

Breathing is not a program; giving your body the nutrients it requires is not a program; sleep is not a program. This book IS NOT a program. If you want to raise my stress levels really fast, refer to it as that. Programs, diets, and pills are the problem with our obesity- and chronic-disease-ridden healthcare system. Programs are short-lived. Programs have end dates. Programs restrict you and handcuff you, making you crave "bad things" more. How long do you want to be healthy? Then it's time to de-program.

What you want are habits. The habits of a healthy person are the secret sauce. With habit changes, you'll get healthy and lose weight instead of losing weight to get healthy. You won't deal with sickness as it comes—you'll beat it before it shows up. You'll create energy each day with movement instead of waiting for it to occasionally surge. It takes as little as 21 days to establish a habit.

Achieving new habits and positively re-enforcing them is a magical moment where healthy becomes your lifestyle. So if we are starting with the end in mind, then the end game is your understanding, living, and WANTING to give your body all that it needs to thrive as your new Livingood Daily Lifestyle. Doesn't that sound amazing? That you can get to a point that you would prefer the veggies over the cheesecake. You'd prefer more rest than binge-watching Netflix. That you would WANT to exercise instead of hit snooze.

How do we get people over and over again to predictably get results and overcome all levels of disease? We follow a formula. I was a biochemistry minor in college, and to create a solution we followed an exact, measured-out formula, one that was studied, scientific, and obedient to the laws of nature. If we did not follow a formula, we risked failing and blowing things up in the lab. There is no need to experiment with your health. For over a decade, I have led thousands of people, done and still do exhaustive research, spent thousands of personal dollars, and experimented on myself. I lived the worst-case scenario with my dad and saw him prevail. This formula is tested, researched, and proven.

Which diet, which workout, what I think about oatmeal or alkaline water, etc, comes later. Those are tools, like the beaker, scale, Bunsen burner, and stir stick. The formula is what gives us the results. So before you go making things complicated or thinking that you've heard all this before, go to work on the substances that make the formula work. Just follow the steps we will unpack in the coming chapters to get your solution.

Step 1 of the Livingood Daily Formula is what we covered in the last chapter. You MUST change, and change now. It doesn't mean you may not still be uncertain or still scared. You might be such a mess you may not have any idea where to start. We will cover the steps, but the most important thing is that you DECIDE "I MUST CHANGE". You may be thinking, "I don't think I can do it, Dr. Livingood." "I don't know if I have that in me."

YES! YES, you do. We are going to USE all that past failure to learn what not to do and free you from the shackles of programs and diets to focus on what you can do. What you MUST do.

Talkback to that "yakety-yak" voice in your head. Interrupt it. A pattern interrupt is exactly what it needs. "Shut your mouth, you unhealthy, negative voice!" I talk back to mine—I even named them!

Don't be a Barry or Sally.

Have you ever seen the movie Inside Out? Well, being a dad of 3, I get to watch my fair share of kids' movies and my favorites are from Disney and Pixar. Inside Out is a catchy story about the multiple voices inside a little girl's head and how they work together and drive her emotions. It is quite funny and very cute. If you have kids or grandkids, it's worth a watch. I think it beautifully sums up what is going on in most of our heads. It's like there are multiple little people up there pulling levers. Meet two of mine.

First, there is Sally. Sally is the whiny resistor that wants to find why something is wrong and disagree, instead of finding the

25

good and making progress. She'll find a reason to complain about everything! "Pipe down, Sally!"

Then there is Barry. Barry might as well be Sally's lazy, "stuck-in-his-ways" husband. He's got a deep Southern voice in my head, maybe because I live in the South. Oh, he's into fitness alright—fittin' nis' whole burger in his mouth! He's always saying, "I'm gonna die o' somethin', so who cares, Doc!" He thinks he eats enough vegetables because he eats potatoes. It seems you can't tell Barry nothin'!

Those voices need to be put into their place almost daily! However, you can use them to strengthen yourself when you learn how to talk back to them. You may say negative things to yourself, but that's not you who are. Impose your will and dictate your own healthy narrative. Snap out of that unhealthy thinking. The same level of thinking that created the problem won't solve it. We have to elevate our thinking and [emotional] state to create change.

Your problems may never completely go away, but you can lift yourself above them and get a fresh new perspective on them. Climb the mountain a bit and look down on your problems from a new vantage point. You may not be able to change your height, genetics, past failures, addictions, or looks. You CAN change how you respond to those situations, as well as your perspective of them.

Building health is going to pull this positivity out of you. Climbing the mountain can be a ton of fun! Imagine how much your life changes when you feel strong, have endless energy, and look forward to each day. It will happen when you desire the outcome of health more than the short-term pleasure of food and laziness. You CAN do that. I am 100% certain of it because you hold the keys: your choices. It's as simple as stopping your brain when it wants the old poor choices and rewiring it to want better choices.

If you find yourself still consistently making the bad choices or giving in to "Sally" and "Barry," then you are simply making the choice in the wrong state of mind. You are NOT alone. A good state of mind drives good choices, but a lot of us still live in anxious, fearful, negative mental environments (states).

If I were to ask you to work out with me after a long day of work when you are exhausted, or in the middle of the night while you are sleeping, or right after you watch the news, what are the chances you would say yes? Slim to none. But if I were to put your favorite song on, ask you to list 10 things that are awesome in your life right now, and ask you to work out with me at your most freed-up time of day, what are the chances you would say yes? Nearly 100%! Same person, same workout, but a different state. If you don't believe me, just start laughing out loud right now and watch what happens to your state and how you feel. Try it. Start laughing!

Become your head of state.

Learn to trigger your body out of "I'm not feeling it" to "I want it!" There are four FAST ways to do this:
1. Music – Some days you need the music, some days you need the lyrics!
2. Encouraging Groups and Friends – If the people around you are dragging you down, then get around better people. Social Media has made this easier than ever.
3. Motivational Teachings and Shows – Listen daily! I do several, or many of these a week for our community for

this exact reason. Shut off the radio or Hulu, and turn on something to make you better. Garbage in, garbage out. Good in, good out. What are you putting in?

4. Planned Scheduling – You plan to fail when you fail to plan. If it's not scheduled, it's not happening. The MOST important appointments and events in your life are what you schedule. Isn't your health worth putting on the calendar?

This is the first habit to commit to, as it feeds all others. We help people do this every day in our Livingood Daily Challenges. We know if the state holds the key to making choices that create habits, then we get you in to an environment to set you up to succeed. Environment matters. You could be the fastest runner in the world, but if I put you in mud, you won't fare well. If you don't have a good environment, don't let that be an excuse, Sally. Find a better one. Online challenge groups give you that encouraging and empowering state no matter where you live. Go to *www.livingooddaily.com* to learn more.

Can you begin to see why so many people fail on programs and diets? First, there cannot be an ounce of "I should." We have to get to the point of decision: "I MUST change my health, or I am going to end up like my parents or a statistic. Plus, I have a purpose in the world and God isn't done with me yet!" Next, make a state and environment change to set yourself up to want to choose the better choices. The tools I give you for nutrition, fitness, or stress relief won't matter if you don't know how and why they work. If I hand you a screwdriver and you don't know how and why to use the screwdriver, then the tool might as well be a paperweight. So now that you are committed to change and we have established you as Head of State, let's begin to overhaul the health department.

What is health?

If you really want to achieve it, then you've got to know what health is in the first place. How do you know if you're healthy? What a question that is! Honestly, how do you really, truly judge if you're healthy or not?

The average person would say they judge their health based on how they feel; in other words, how you felt when you woke up this morning—if you were able to walk, if you were able to move, if you got to work, if you felt okay, and if you weren't all congested or run-down or hurting, then you assume you're healthy.

The second way a lot of people judge is how they look. We've been sold magazine covers and books and self-help guides with people who have muscles and abs and an image on the cover, and we assume that if we look a certain way, then we must be healthy.

I'm not going to argue that physical fitness is not an important aspect of being healthy, but explain how someone like Jim Fixx, who invented jogging (the concept of running to be healthy) back in the 1950s, died while jogging at age 52 from heart failure. The Biggest Loser host, Bob Harper, is another example who had a massive heart attack at age 51.

The third way that people try to analyze their health is by having tests done. There is merit and there is importance in testing and identifying conditions via blood work and diagnostic imaging. If the test comes back positive, what do you already have? The disease. So, these are disease tests, not health tests.

Could you look good, feel good, and pass the physical, but still have heart disease or cancer? For sure, it happens thousands of times per day.

The World Health Organization defines health as 100% functioning and healing. On the World Health Organization's website, it says health is a state of complete physical, mental, and social well-being, not merely the absence of disease or infirmity.[20] The leader on health in the world says it's not feeling and looking good—it's all about function.

100% functioning and healing is the definition of health, which means 0% functioning and healing is the definition of death. Let's avoid that for you at all costs.

Everyone, including you reading this book, is somewhere in between the scale of 0% to 100% functioning and healing. If your heart, for example, is functioning at 100%, it's impossible to get heart disease; also, if your immune system is functioning at 100%, it is impossible to get cancer. If your body and organs are functioning at 100%, then you are at your full health potential.

It works the same way as light and darkness. There is no such thing as darkness. It's just a lack of light. There's really no such thing as disease. It is just a lack of health. There are names we attach to a lack of health issues, i.e., diseases. The problem is always the same, though; lack of health. When you reach 100% of your full health potential, you are healthy.

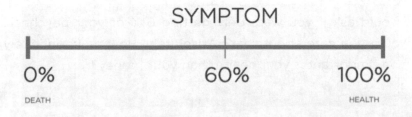

Research shows that you have to get down to around 60% functioning and healing before you have your first symptom and actually know you're unhealthy.[21,22,23,24] That means you do not know you have a problem in most areas of your body, especially in your organs, until they are functioning at 60% or below. We easily understand this with a blocked artery. An artery can be 99% blocked before you actually feel the dysfunction.

I recently spoke to a group of doctors and nurses at a hospital in the nephrology unit. I asked the nephrologist, "At what percentage can you feel your kidneys dysfunction?" I told him research shows that your kidneys have to be all the way down to 40% function before you can actually feel that the kidneys have a problem.[25]

He replied, "It's more like 10%!"

You can lose 90% of the function of your kidneys and not feel it! Yet, most people judge their health based on what? How they feel.

So, if you are walking around only getting 60% of the function of an organ, would you want to know that? When would you want to know that? You don't even feel it until it gets to that point, which means you could be sitting at 61%, and guess what? You don't know that you even have a problem.

I would ask if you were only getting 61% of your paycheck, would you care about that? Absolutely. How much infinitely more important is your health than your money?

Your money cannot buy your health back. If that were the case, then Steve Jobs never would have passed away.

———

He was worth over $20 billion, which means your health and your body (which he couldn't buy back) are worth $20 billion or more!

Symptoms start showing up around 60%. When your blood pressure is high or your cholesterol is off, or your blood sugar is high, or you are depressed, or your thyroid is off, or you have migraines, these symptoms show up at 60%. There are three ways to approach symptoms.

Option One: Ignore the symptoms.

The first approach, typically taken by men, is to flat-out do what with your health? Ignore it. You ignore your health until you're forced to do something about it. Why wait to lose your health, and then take care of it? When the pain is great enough? When it ails you and keeps you from doing something? When an organ shuts down? We ignore our health until we have symptoms and keep ignoring it once we get them. Don't ignore your biggest asset; you will always regret that.

Option Two: Cover up the symptoms.

The second approach to our health is to cover up the symptoms. When our vehicles, our bodies, get to 60%, the symptoms occur like check-engine lights on the dashboard, flashing at us and telling us that something is not right, that we need to pop the hood and find out what's going on in this vehicle of ours. But we don't want to deal with it. The second approach, especially in America, is to put a piece of black tape over the check engine light and keep driving.

That's exactly what we are doing with our health symptoms and our own check-engine lights—the warning signs that our bodies are giving us.

The current "sick-care" model says to do what to the symptom? Give it a drug or do surgery because of it. If you simply cover up a symptom with a drug or surgery, you may get relief temporarily; but the second you come off that medication, what happens to the symptom? It comes right back.

You get high blood pressure and are handed a drug for the rest of your life to drive it down to what we call normal. Your cholesterol goes high, and you're stuck on a statin drug for the rest of your life to put it in the normal range. Your blood sugar levels and A1C levels creep up, and you get the diagnosis of being a pre-diabetic or diabetic, so you just take pills to control the condition but never truly address why that warning light came on, thus never discovering what you were doing to the vehicle to cause it to malfunction in the first place.

The other problem with this approach is that every one of those drugs and surgeries comes with deadly side effects. What're the last 30 seconds of a prescription drug commercial? "May cause liver failure, kidney failure, lymphoma, sudden death..." You've heard the sped-up version of this on TV; the average is 70 side effects per pill. 26 If you are taking several drugs at once, it is impossible to know the extent of the effects they are having on your body. People are now taking drugs to counter the side effects of other prescription drugs.

Symptoms are warning signs, so if all you do is ignore your

symptoms or cover them with a drug or surgery, which way on the function scale are you guaranteed to go - toward 100% function or toward 0% function? Toward 0%. And, which way is America's healthcare system going? Toward 0%. We keep getting sicker and sicker and sicker.

In fact, if you go to a doctor in America and do not have a symptom, what does he do to you? He sends you home! We wait for people to get sick, and then we treat those diseases and sicknesses with drugs and surgeries. That's not healthcare, that's sick care! We have a giant sick care system.

We take 75% of the world's drugs while only comprising about 5% of the world's population.[27]

Options one and two above are why we are so sick.

Option Three: Get to the cause.

The third approach is the approach my dad needed. This is the approach I teach my family, the approach I've taken well over 25,000 patients through to help them overcome medications, lose weight, heal from conditions of all kinds that they'd never thought they would heal from. The approach is to focus on taking someone from 37% or 60% or 70%, and move them closer to 100% function—full health and full healing.

How do we actually build health?

If you build health, you get health. If you focus on sickness and disease, you get sickness and disease.

So, how do you and your family move toward a 100% function? How do you move toward a life without medications? How do you move toward a life without diseases and conditions? How do you move toward reaching your full potential? How do you move toward the health of your dreams?

16 YEARS OF MIGRAINES AND 36 DIFFERENT MEDS....GONE!

OFF THYROID MEDS AND SINUS MEDS!

OFF THYROID MED, ALLERGY MED, AND ANTI-INFLAMMATORY MEDS! MOOD HAS IMPROVED AND BACK PAIN IS BETTER!

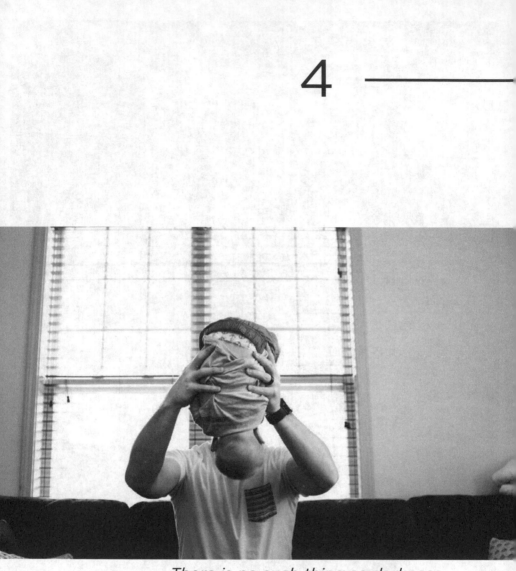

*There is no such thing as darkness,
just lack of light.*

CHAPTER FOUR
REMOVE THE INTERFERENCE

Who is the greatest doctor in the world? A cardiologist from Duke? An oncologist from Mayo Clinic? A researcher from John Hopkins? I'll stop you before you say, "Dr. Livingood." I'll ask you to rethink before you say, "Dr. Oz," "Dr. Phil" or, heaven forbid, "Dr. Seuss." The greatest doctor in the world is reading this book right now—it's you. You are the greatest doctor in the world.

You would say, "Well, Dr. Livingood, I'm not a doctor." Yes, you are. What's happening inside of you right now is so miraculous and so intelligent that no man will ever come close to understanding the power of the doctor that lies within.

How does your body know how to raise its blood pressure and lower it? How does it know how to take food and break it down and absorb it as nutrients, then kick cells and organs and tissue out on the other end? How does it know when to blink?

How does it know when to sleep? How does it know how to do all of these things? That doctor is always on the job, and the day it stops is the day you'll breathe your final breath.

So, there's nothing I can give you in this book—there's no supplement, there's no food, there's no exercise, there's no medication, there's no knife. There's nothing that can come from the outside to give you health. If I give all of these things to a dead person, what happens? Nothing happens. Supplements, food, exercise, and drugs do not do the healing. The only reason they have any beneficial effect is that the doctor on the inside uses them to build health.

Greater is He that is in you
than he that is in the world.
– 1 John 4:4

Don't believe me? Let me show you how powerful you are! [28, 29]
- Nerve impulses in your brain travel as fast as 300 miles an hour. Shake your hand right now. At 170 to 300 miles an hour, that message went from your brain to your hand.
- The brain operates at the same amount of power as a 10-watt light bulb. Well, for some of you, it may be only 5 watts.
- 80% of the brain that you have is water.
- You could remove a large part of your internal organs and you'd still survive.
- The acid in your stomach is strong enough to dissolve razor blades.
- Take a deep breath in. The surface area of your lungs is equivalent to the surface area of a tennis court.
- Pound-for-pound, babies are stronger than oxen.

- Your nose can remember 50,000 different scents.
- Your lungs consist of over 300,000 million capillaries.
- Human bone is 4x stronger than concrete. One cubic inch of your bone can bear a load of 19,000 lbs.
- The focusing muscles of your eyes, looking right now at this book, move about 100,000 times in an average day; that would be the same as walking 50 miles every day for your leg muscles.
- The average human body gives off enough heat in only a half-hour to boil a half-gallon of water.
- The blood vessels in your body, if they were placed end-to-end, would stretch a combined 25,000 miles, long enough to circle the globe.
- You produce enough saliva in your lifetime to fill two swimming pools.
- For those with sweaty feet, your feet have about 500,000 sweat glands and have the ability to produce up to a pint of sweat every day.
- My favorite of them all...make a fist. Your heart is the size of a fist and it weighs about a pound. Go ahead and pump your fist. It produces and pumps about 1.2 million gallons of blood every year. In a 24-hour period of time, your heart gives off enough energy to lift three fully-loaded Greyhound buses off the ground!

That power is in you! Will you put more faith in a drug, injection, surgery, or doctor to heal you than the power of the greatest doctor in the world that lives inside of you?

Every time you need a reminder—when you feel despair, when you feel like you don't have hope, when you feel like you can't heal—just take a look at your hand. Just feel your heartbeat. Just take a deep breath into your lungs. Many people didn't wake up with those things today, but you did—which means the power is alive and well inside of you.

You are the greatest doctor in the world, and the power that's on the inside makes all the difference. That power does not need any help or interference; we're messing it up. If we can remove the interference, the power can go to work.

The power is always on at 100%, but it cannot work if you interfere with it. It's like a faucet turned on wide open. The faucet isn't the problem. The problem occurs when you kink the hose. The water can't get through to water the garden so it can reach its potential. When you remove the interference, healing happens every single time. So, what kinks the hose?

When you get to the cause of the symptoms, you don't need medicine unless there is a crisis. If you also change your lifestyle along the way, you can radically reduce your risk of disease in the first place. Building health—that's real health care. The key lies in the power inside of you!

It's the doctor—it's the power that's on the inside—that makes all the difference, and that power does not need any help—it just needs no interference. The problem is that you are messing it up. Come on! Are you messing up your health right now? Remove the interference and you'll heal.

If I gave you a paper cut on your finger right now, what would it do? Hurt, yes. And then it would bleed, but, eventually, it would clot and heal over the next coming days or week. Yes? You wouldn't just bleed out and that would be it. Your cut would heal, which would mean your healing mechanism is working!

So, why aren't your headaches healing? Why isn't your thyroid healing? Why isn't your digestive system healing? Why isn't that lower back pain healing? Why isn't the numbness and tingling healing? Why isn't your reproductive system healing? Why isn't your heart healing? Why aren't all these other conditions healing, when your healing mechanism is working?

Something is interfering with the doctor on the inside from doing his or her job. If you can find the cause of the interference, your body can heal, no matter what the condition is. The key is removing the interference.

If you focus on and treat sickness and disease, you get sickness and disease! If you focus on and build health, you get health. This fundamental principle guides any practical steps you take to live good daily.

We need to establish where you are interfering with your health, and we'll take massive action to remove that interference. There are three main causes of interference with the doctor on the inside; they all start with *T*, so it's pretty nice teaching.

If you can remove the interference, you get to experience real health.

1. Thoughts

Is stress the main thing that's bogging down your health? Is the constant cortisol taking its toll on your joints or digestive system? What about the function of your organs? Is the stress of your brain just wearing you out? Practically, removing thought interference involves dealing with negativity, emotional strain, depression, state, and stress. All these physiologically interfere with and damage the healing inside your body.

Mentally, we carry weight around on a daily basis; all kinds of thoughts affect how our body works. Negative thoughts pull us away from health, lower our overall state, and hinder our body's ability to function and heal properly as intended. The more connected we can get with those thoughts, control them, and make them positive, the more it will increase the healing inside of our body.

2. Toxins

The more toxicity that gets into your body, the more interference the doctor on the inside experiences, making it unable to do its job.

The two main sources of toxicity in today's world are food and lack of movement. So, the two main goals are to fix your fitness and to fix your food.

I wonder as you read this right now—do you know that what you're eating is greatly affecting your health? Do you know you need to clean up your diet? Are you succumbing to the constant pull of temptations of food? Do you hate to exercise? Maybe you don't have time to exercise. If this is you, then fixing your food and fitness will be the main focus.

Toxins build up in our body from the things we eat and are exposed to daily as Americans. We take four billion prescription drugs a year. Ten thousand toxins are used in the processes of making our foods. Fifty thousand chemicals are used to process products that we purchase, and these are in your home on a daily basis. The more toxins that are allowed into your body, the more interference to the healing power inside is created.

3. Traumas

Trauma may be the number-one missing piece in health care today. Trauma to your body damages the tissue (athletics, posture, accidents, falls, etc.). Do you have damaged joints that prevent you from working out? Ailments that cause you pain? Traumas like these—especially to your spine—block the healing power of your nervous system from getting into your body; these traumas build up over a lifetime and interfere with real health.

These three *T*'s are the cause of interference in our bodies. When you remove interference, the body heals every single time.

Treat Your Body Like a Plant

My wife and I are horrible at taking care of plants; most of them do not survive in our house. What are the things a plant needs in order to survive?—water, sunlight, soil, and carbon dioxide. If the plant were withering, you would remove the interference and give it one of those necessary things: you'd move it into the sun, give it water, or even talk to it. You might change the soil or give it fertilizer, and the plant would be restored to life. You wouldn't cut a leaf off and rub aspirin on it; you would remove the interference, and the healing in the plant would restore it back to new!

Your body works the same way: give it what it needs, remove what it doesn't, and it will be healthy!

There is no such thing as darkness, just lack of light. If

something is interfering with the light, uncover it, and the light shines again. The sun is always shining; you just need to move the clouds.

There is no such thing as disease,
just lack of health.

I know we refer to common conditions in medical terms so that we know to call the lump "breast cancer" or the sneezing "allergies," but it is all just lack of health. If health existed at 100%, then diseases would not exist at all.

In the last 3 chapters, we have been laying out a formula, The Livingood Daily Formula.

1. We must change, and change now. No more diets, no more programs, and no more pills. It's time to get to the cause and develop lifelong habits.
2. Become your head of state. Set yourself up to make the daily choices to build health.
3. Remove the interference. In the next few chapters, we will follow the 5 fixes to remove the interference.

Steps 4 and 5 of the master formula are coming, but it's time to get practical. In the following 6 chapters, I will break down the most simple and powerful health changes you can make. This information will lay the groundwork for the Livingood Daily Challenge, where we will help you apply the information, turn it into knowledge, and establish habits to change your life.

FREEDOM = OFF AN ENTIRE BAG OF DRUGS!

OFF REFLUX, DEPRESSION, SLEEP, MIGRAINE, AND PAIN MEDS! OFF 5 MEDS!

LOW BACK PAIN, NECK PAIN AND SKIN ISSUES GONE!

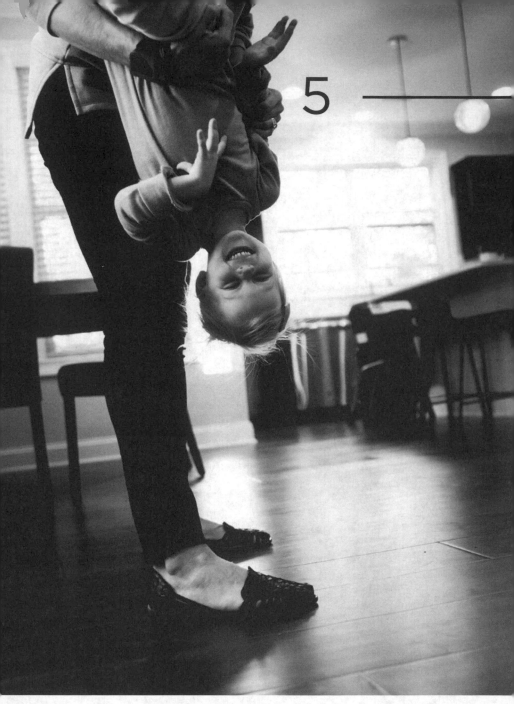

5

As a man thinkith, so is he.

CHAPTER FIVE
FIX YOUR FOCUS

The first *T* of interference is *thoughts—*your thinking. The main part of this is stress. Is stress bogging down your health? Is the constant cortisol taking its toll on your joints, your digestive system, the function of your organs? Is the stress of your brain just wearing you out? If that's you, then this is the main *T* to get you going.

Thoughts are also the way that you look at health care. I've just spent the entire first part of this book changing the way you think, helping you start to see what actual health is, in order to see that we don't have a healthcare system—we have a sick-care system. If you don't want to be sick, then you need to get out of that system and start thinking differently. Change your state and fix your focus.

Let's jump into the stress side of things. You can deploy very simple tactics to deal with stress. Here's the big tagline:

You cannot manage stress.

_____

It's impossible. Stop trying to! Stuff is going to go wrong today, this week, this month, and this year. Unforeseen events come up and cause the most stress.

I mean, who can predict a flat tire? Who can predict someone going down at work and leaving all the stress on you? Who can predict a sick child? These stressful events come out of nowhere, so you can neither control nor manage them.

Do you have children? You can't manage stress! I have three kids myself. If you have kids, you understand that life can be unpredictable and stressful.

You can't manage stress, but you can manage your focus, your response to stress. You can manage the way you approach every situation, every day. Each situation can be seen as an opportunity, or it can be seen as an obstacle. You can approach the stressful situation with a calm, sound mind, or with anger, offense, and worry.

If I were to give you the simplest 2-step teaching on stress— how to deal with it, how to have less of it, and how to reduce the negative impact it may have on you—I would start by teaching you about perspective.

As you read this book right now, I want you to take a deep breath in and then breathe all the way out.

_____

You woke up today. Do you know how many people didn't?

Do you know how many people took the last breath they'll ever take yesterday, or during their sleep last night?

If you're like me, you woke up in one of the greatest countries in the world, with all sorts of freedom and opportunities. You won the lottery if you were born in or live in America right now, because of all the opportunities that you have. You could be in much worse parts of the world, with severely limited resources, stuck in an area that you'd never get out of.

Did you wake up with a roof over your head today? You didn't wake up on the streets, right? Then, you've got a lot going for you.

Did you get in a car today? Do you know how many people don't have one of those? You get to transport yourself around. Did you go to a job? Do you know how many millions of people (in our country alone) don't have one of those?

The point is that there's so much more going right for you today than what's going wrong for you today, but all you've been taught to focus on is what's going wrong. Before you even rolled out of bed, a lot of good was happening in your world and in your life, and there's so much to be thankful for. So, the main remedy for stress is gratitude—everyone can cultivate more gratitude.

The best remedy for stress is gratitude.

The first thing I have trained my brain to do every morning is to smile because I woke up again, and then I immediately start listing my "grats." What if you woke up each morning surprised!? Like WHOA! I get another one! Haha, it makes me laugh just thinking of starting every day that way.

As a simple tactic, spend a few minutes every morning of your day, every day, thinking about what you're thankful for—your spouse, your children, your house, the things that you have in your life...your purpose, your job, your co-workers, your pets, your eyes, your lungs, your heart...anything that you're thankful for. The more specific you are, the more powerful you'll feel. Your "grats" are gifts that are not guaranteed tomorrow. As the saying goes, that's why they call today the "present."

Fix your focus. Be grateful for everything you have in your life. When you approach your day with this frame of mind, it just makes your problems and the stress you face much less of a burden; however, it doesn't mean problems aren't going to happen.

I know you may be reading this and going through a very challenging situation in your life, but I challenge you, every time those stressful moments come up, to go right back to gratitude and focus your mind on all the good things that are going on right in that moment, not just the bad things.

I could take you to some areas of this world that would make your stressful, taxing situation look really small in the grand scheme of things. Many of the things we call problems and major stressors are not really that big a deal.

Losing a loved one or having something happen to a child or a spouse—those are stressful situations. We've gotten to the point, especially in America, that we treat everyday stresses as if one of our loved ones is dying or has just been diagnosed with a terminal illness. Don't do that to yourself every day. Put things in perspective; most stuff is just not that big a deal. Focus—you have a ton to be grateful for.

Take a "smoke break."

Step 2 to reduce stress is to strengthen your brakes. Inside your body is a sympathetic nervous system that controls the "stress" or "fight" response of your body. This is like your accelerator. The other nervous system you have is the parasympathetic nervous system that controls the "healing" or "flight" response of your body. These are like your brakes.

Your stress response was designed to protect you from a bear in the woods or a rattlesnake crossing your path. Your rest response is meant for digesting food, healing, reproducing, and sleeping. Let me explain with a near-death experience...

About 7 years ago, I was rushing across town on an errand, 3 hours before a flight I had to catch. I was flying back to Iowa for my wife's family "Thanksmas," our annual gathering combining Thanksgiving and Christmas.

"Thanksmas" was a real boost to the parasympathetic system—4 days cut off from work to play, laugh, and take lots of naps in a small town in "heaven." (If you have seen the movie *Field of Dreams*, you understand why I refer to Iowa as that!) We would completely de-stress and power-up the parasympathetic nervous system. We would run an easy turkey-trot, watch lots of football, take long naps, laugh, and of course digest loads of healthy and not-so-healthy food. Thanksgiving dinner is my favorite! I couldn't wait for the ultimate family weekend, and neither could my stress system.

I still had to finish this errand, but I needed gas. I whipped into the BP gas station and filled up. I checked my emails while I waited for the tank to click full and then was on my way. I drove past the giant tanker parked halfway in the entrance of the small gas station and turned onto the road back towards the clinic. WHAM! An 18-wheeler smashed the front of my truck. My immediate "stress" response probably saved my life as I managed to swerve at the last second, or that thing would have been in my lap! Needless to say, my cortisol, stress, and sympathetic nervous system were through the roof as I came to a halt. I got clearance from the vehicle and thanked God for not a single scratch on me or the other driver.

The next wave of stress set in. "Marv" was hurting. Marv (so-named by my best friends) was the Toyota Tacoma my dad and mom had gotten me at age 16. Not only was I now facing a big police report, an insurance game, and a huge bill, I also didn't have a ride. These were the days before Uber! I had to get back across town, or I was going to miss my flight and "Thanksmas"! My sympathetic nervous system was going wild! It turned out my wife ended up being my "Uber driver," Marv found a tow truck and lived to drive another day, and "Thanksmas" turned out pretty darn good, all things considered. I was able to drive—pun intended—my stress levels down and actually enjoy the holiday.

We now live in a day and age where our bodies are under constant stress—the kind we are meant to experience after being in a car accident or chased by a wild bear. Your stress system gets this kind of stimulation just sitting at work rushing to beat a deadline, racing your kids around to events, stewing over the news, arguing with a friend over politics, skipping sleep to watch Game of Thrones. High- and low-grade stress, worry, and anxiousness for some are NON-STOP. Our accelerators are stuck.

Some of these stress inducers, as we mentioned, you cannot control. You can, however, strengthen your brakes. If you cannot avoid the activities accelerating your stress, then you must implement techniques to strengthen your brakes, to briefly slow down your system and organs and fire your healing parasympathetic nervous system. How do you do this? Breathing.

Long, deep breaths have been shown to regulate your parasympathetic nervous system and strengthen your brakes. The technique is called paced or boxed, breathing.

This breathing improves your heart rate variability by stimulating the nerve that controls the brakes for all of your vital organs. By stimulating your parasympathetic nervous system, you lower your blood pressure, aid digestion, increase immunity, increase longevity, and lower your risk for heart attacks and cancer—just by proper breathing.[30]

Here's how:
Paced Breathing: Take a 5-second deep breath in and at least a 5-second deep breath out. Continue for 2 minutes and crank up the healthy oxygen into your system.

Boxed Breathing: Take a 4-second deep breath in, hold for 4 seconds, and take at least a 4-second breath out. Repeat for 2 minutes.

I call it "Nature's Smoke Break"—some call it smelling the roses or blowing out the candles; but whatever you call it, research shows it works. If smokers can reduce their stress with a toxin multiple times a day, you can reduce yours with a walk and some breathing. Combine steps 1 and 2 and you have a simple, yet powerful technique to strengthen your brakes and decrease your stress. Take several of "nature's smoke breaks" throughout your day. Go for a 2-5 minute walk with no technology, put a smile on your face, FOCUS on what you are grateful for, and breathe.

Take a breathing break, skip the cigarette, and pump the brakes! Your heart, anxiety, organs, and body will love you for it. You will find that this life really is amazing if you just take a minute to soak it in.

Bonus: Sleep and Stress Aids

In the age of depression, anxiety, and stress, I would rather see someone try an herb before resorting to a toxic drug to deal with stress. Getting to the cause is always first, so commit to your breathing and gratitude training first. If you still have cortisol you can't avoid, here are a few of my favorite tactics and herbs to support your system.

Sleep! Consider these facts:
- 50 to 70 million Americans struggle with some type of sleep disorder.
- 50% of Americans deal with some level of snoring or have a family member that deals with it. I don't have a magical solution for snoring, but a lot of it is related to sleep apnea.
- 25 million Americans deal with sleep apnea.
- 5% of people get drowsy while driving. This is scary, by the way, so rest really matters.
- At least 100,000 medical errors happen every single year, and many of them are from sleep deprivation.
- 8% of people reported unintentionally falling asleep at some point during the day–a form of narcolepsy or an effect of sleep apnea.

If you don't rest, you can't be your best. Nighttime TV, phone use, excessive eating, or reading fiction books just do not add much value to your life. You can still do some, but set a time, cut it off, and get some rest. Tomorrow needs you rested, de-stressed, and ready to seize the opportunities.

Are you restless? Are you waking up a lot? No matter how much sleep you get, you're still tired when you wake up in the morning? There are many different variables when it comes to not sleeping well, and I'm going to give you 9 simple hacks that you can use to help with sleep. They are real, simple things you can implement this evening.

Here are the simple hacks to get down to the bottom of it.

- Technology. It's a good friend. It enables us to do a lot of things, but it greatly interrupts sleep. The only thing that should be happening in your bed is sleep, right? (If you're married, maybe another thing, but that's a whole other topic.) This means no TV. You should not have your phone in bed. No technology should be happening there. You've really got to protect that bedroom and that bed. You have to protect that area so that you're not allowing too many things to interfere with what your body needs to do–get rest.

  Research shows that your nervous system speeds up when you sleep. Every other system goes down. That's what heals you and helps you recover from the day that you just had. Technology interferes with that, whether it's the screen of a TV that lulls you to sleep or the screen of your phone. Technology interferes with the brain and the activity that it needs to do–get you into a deep sleep so your body can heal.

- Environment. Analyze the room that you actually sleep in. You can look at a couple of different things:

1. Light. I remember back when I really started to understand this better and protect the sleep that my wife and I got, we hung a big curtain so we could make the room really dark. We did that in our children's room as well, because there were lots of lights shining in from street lights outside of our apartment. Now we have shades and blinds that help block the light. You want it to be very dark.

2. Temperature. Keeping it as low as 65 degrees in your bedroom helps your body fall asleep faster because your core temperature actually decreases at night. If the room is already cold, it helps your body get there faster. If you take a long time to fall asleep, turn the temperature down, and that will help you.

- Sleep Schedule. Depending on your career, this might be difficult. But having a regular, regimented sleep schedule, especially Monday through Friday (or following your workweek) is very important. This means that you should go to bed around the same time every evening, and get up around the same time every morning. The further you get away from that, the more it messes up the rhythm of your body and the schedule that it becomes accustomed to.

For example, if during the week you go to bed at 11 p.m. and you get up at 6 a.m., and then on the weekend you sleep in till 9 a.m., you oftentimes feel groggy. Maybe some of you are thinking, "I would LOVE to try to sleep in because it never happens." When you try to do it, it can actually work against you because it's messing with your body's current sleep rhythm. Working with that rhythm is extremely important.

- Diet. If you're eating large meals close to bedtime, and

toxic, high sugar, not-so-good-for-you meals close to bedtime, that's really going to interrupt your sleep pattern. From a physiological standpoint, your body is trying to process all that food, spending a lot of energy on digestion, instead of allowing you to go to sleep to heal your body. Late, unhealthy meals can also cause digestive problems like an upset stomach, acid reflux, and heartburn.

To help remedy nighttime indigestion, you could try apple cider vinegar, 1-2 tbsp. Before or after your meal. Also, because of where the stomach sits, sleeping on your left side would allow your stomach to digest food a lot better, as opposed to the right.

Watch your caffeine intake later in the day, as well. Obviously, it's going to keep you more wide awake into the evening. Forcing your body to do that really throws off the sleep rhythm.

- Exercise. Studies show that exercise does help a person sleep better. If you currently exercise, but have sleep struggles, consider hanging the time that you exercise. If you are a morning exerciser and are not sleeping well, you may try to move the exercise to the evening. If you're an evening or afternoon exerciser and you're not sleeping well, you may try to move the exercise to the morning. The response and the impact that exercise has on your body can greatly impact how your body rests. So you may just need to change the timing.

- Supplements. There are a couple of supplements that you could try if you are really not getting sleep. However, I would warn you that you should not rely on a natural supplement. That's just like any dependence on sleep medication. There are side effects of sleep medications. In the long term, there will be side effects with having natural substances that put you to sleep each night. If you want to start with a supplement, skip to the cortisol section below to focus on the cause, which is more than likely to affect your stress levels and diet.

- Spinal Exercises. A lot of people cannot sleep because they're uncomfortable. The frame of their body is not in the right position, whether on their back, side, or stomach. If the spine is in a bad position, the body can't rest the way it's designed to. We discuss solutions to this in the Fix Your Frame Chapter.

- Epsom Salt Bath. Epsom salt is fantastic for detoxing the body. It is high in the relaxing mineral magnesium and a great detoxifier. I highly recommend it to pull out toxins, especially from the skin. It will dilate the blood vessels near the skin and flush those toxins out. Your body will respond by being very relaxed, drowsy, and sometimes even a little dizzy. With the Epsom salt bath's heat and blood vessel dilation, it's a great thing to do right before going to sleep. You're detoxing the system, opening up the blood vessels, and putting your body into more of a rest mode. Just be careful standing up, because you may be a little light-headed. Try a cup of Epsom salt in a bath or a dose of 200-400mg of magnesium before bed. It's lights out!

- Go to Bed Earlier. Most people do not have a "getting up early" problem, they have a "going to bed early" problem. From a cortisol standpoint, when you go to bed at a later time, you're interfering with your cortisol arch, and the pattern that it's supposed to follow during the day.

Your cortisol is your stress hormone, and it happens to peak early in the morning. Research shows that the later you go to bed, the more you're actually allowing that cortisol spike to happen earlier.

Have you ever experienced this–you wake up and you're almost in a panic-type scenario? Or you had a dream, and you wake up stressed out because of the dream? Am I the only one? That is the worst thing ever! You're sleeping and getting stressed out! I've always just thought, "Well, it's just the luck of the draw of my dream."

What is actually happening is that the cortisol levels are spiking too early. They're not waiting for you to get up, but are spiking at 4 am or earlier. A lot is tied to when you go to bed and properly taking care of these cortisol levels. If this is you—regularly waking up anxious in the mornings, then address your cortisol.

Cortisol, your stress hormone, is produced in your adrenal glands, so the simple support of those organs is a great start. Adaptogenic herbs have been shown to be a great tool to de-stress. Ashwagandha has the biggest impact, lowering cortisol up to a whopping 32%.[30] Ginseng and Rhodiola are other herbs that have been shown to restore normal patterns of eating and sleeping after stress, lower mental and physical fatigue, and protect against oxidative stress, heat stress, radiation, and exposure to toxic chemicals.

The International Society of Sports Nutrition in 2010 published a study showing that when you take 2400 milligrams of Omega-3 you can actually decrease the cortisol spike that happens in the morning. Another supplement you can look at is B5. High levels of B5 have been shown to reduce your cortisol and your stress levels, especially for that morning spike. Getting proper vitamin

C allows for proper adrenal function, which decreases the chance of that early morning cortisol spike so you don't wake up anxious. Eighty percent of your vitamin C is actually stored in your adrenal glands. I regularly take a dose of vitamin C in the afternoon for my cortisol and immune system. For more of a calming effect, herbal teas like chamomile are great in the evening. Other agents to calm the system are gamma-aminobutyric acid (GABA) and L-theanine which have been shown to combat anxiety and relax the system from fear and stress. These could be used anytime during the day when anxiety persists.

Just remember, stress and anxiety are a programmable response to our environment. Every form of it can, at a minimum, be improved. Training your brain to stop the stress and focus on the good is like training a muscle. If you don't use it, you lose it. Start giving your brain workouts today.

If you have health and your family has health today, then you have a lot! If you have breath in your lungs, then you are winning! You don't have to spend another day stressing if you choose not to; you can choose to be thankful regardless of what this life throws at you.

Accept what life has given you, be grateful for all of it, and focus your thoughts on progressing as a human. Building health is the only way to get healthy, so let's fix the next cause of interference.

IBS NO LONGER!
HEADACHE FREE AND
CAN WORK OUT AGAIN!

CUT BLOOD PRESSURE MED IN
HALF, PAIN IS GONE, AND LOST
40 POUNDS AND 4 INCHES!

STOPED SPINAL DECAY!

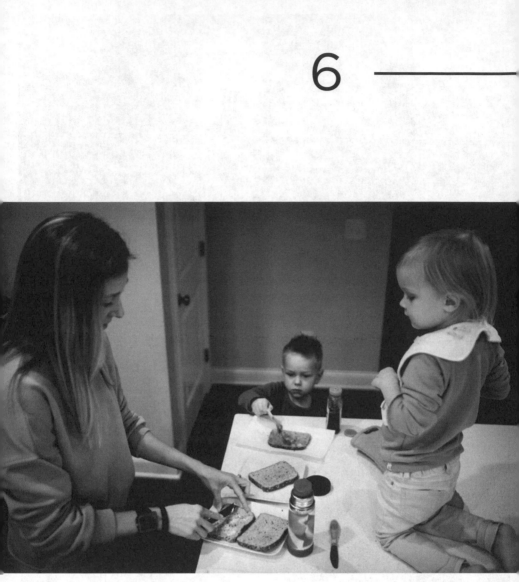

"One must eat to live, not live to eat."
- Moliere.

CHAPTER SIX

FIX YOUR FOOD

Is nutrition the area of health that Is affecting you the most? Has food become an idol? Everything we do now is based around food—unhealthy food—especially on holidays, gatherings, work time, date nights, and vacations. During the holidays, the mealtime discussions revolve around what we are making for the next meal! Before church services, we have food, in the middle of services we have food, and after church services we have food. Everything we do is based around food.

We can get food on the go, we can get food at midnight, we can get food delivered to us, we can get food at all times in all quantities, in endless amounts. Overseas countries and people often struggle with lack—lack of clean water, lack of food, and lack of healthcare. In America, we struggle with excess—too much food, too many toxins, too much laziness.

I really believe food has become an idol, so nutrition is one big area we're going to tackle, and we keep it very simple in this book. Eat real food versus fake food. To put it another way, eat food by God, versus food by man.

The more food you can eat that God has put here for you to enjoy (foods in their purest form) the healthier you are; however, the more man processes it, interferes with it, and changes it, the worse it gets. Fake food (food by man) can be extremely toxic. Your body has some amazing detoxifiers in your liver, kidneys, and digestive system, but it can only handle so much.

This supersedes all "diet" approaches. It doesn't matter if you are vegetarian, carnivore, paleo, keto, etc.—just eat real food! You can be vegetarian and still eat pizza, chips, and beer! You can be keto or carnivore, and load up on toxic bacon and artificial sweeteners. Real food is the one requirement for any of those ways of eating to be healthy.

The Death of Dieting

For 21 days, or until you reach your goal, I'm going to challenge you to eat only real food and give your system a complete break. You'll do this through a couple of simple steps. I don't want to focus on just what you can't eat. I'll never tell you not to eat food ever again, because you're just going to crave that food even more. It's like telling you not to eat Oreos, so you tuck them in the highest cupboard in the kitchen, but in the middle of the night, you're going to crave them and you're going to be scrambling to get to that bag of Oreos.

First, in order to enjoy those things that are bad for us, but not let them control or harm us, we do vacation days. Vacation days are when you can eat what you really enjoy. For my wife, it's pizza; for me, it's a good dessert. When we have those days, we always make sure that we do a workout in the morning. We prepare our bodies, i.e., we eat well during the week, so that when we indulge and enjoy some of those bad-for-us foods, we don't have to feel guilty about it, because we know our health is still on track.

The problem for so many of us is that every day is a vacation day!

Every meal is a vacation meal. When you treat yourself over and over and over again, it's not a treat; it's an expense;—an expense on your pocket and —an expense on your health. So for that reason, you would do well to abstain from using vacation meals until you hit your goals or at least for 21 days.

You have to completely cut yourself off from that way of living and those habits for a 21-day period of time, and then you can use that momentum to establish real lifetime eating changes while adding the vacation-day concept to enjoy your favorites. It's time to re-establish your relationship with food, especially if you are addicted. EVERY bad food you love can be replaced with something healthy, or you can find a way to make it healthy yourself. For now, over the next few weeks, it's time to buckle down.

When I start messing with food, a lot of people are quick to get frustrated and angry because they focus on how hard it is. Let me change your perspective once again on this. Losing your health is hard, but, comparatively, a 21-day challenge is easy! When my dad had his chest sawed open and a pig's valve put in—that was hard. When my dad lost his hearing for good—that was hard. Eating healthy is EASY! When you have a big enough "why" to experience real health, then the "how" is easy. Let's dive into the "how."

So, we have to completely take you off, "cold turkey" and keep you off so many of those processed foods, snacks, fried foods, and bad-for-you drinks that you enjoy on a daily basis. If you want to get someone off alcohol, you've got to completely cut him or her off "cold turkey." If you want to get someone off sugar, you've got to cut him or her off "cold turkey" and replace it with healthy fuel.

Here are the Five C's of fixing your food:
1. *Cut the Sugar.*
2. *Crank Up the Fat.*
3. *Clean Up the Protein.*
4. *Care About Nutrients.*
5. *Curb Your Consumption.*

1. Cut the Sugar.

Research shows that the average American eats around 130 pounds of sugar every year! Compare that to the turn of the 19th century in America, when an individual ate less than 20 pounds a year. 38 Sugar is in everything! Why? It tastes sweeter, so you eat more. Food companies know this, and they are exploiting this all the way to the grave. Sugar is an anti-nutrient—not only does it harm you, but it also takes up space for needed nutrients. It all has to go now!

The first initial response I get to that statement is, "I don't eat that much sugar, Dr. Livingood." Yes, you do. They are hidden and you just don't yet know how to find them—which foods constitute or turn into sugar. Understand that I'm writing this book right now to a world of sugar addicts. When you try to tell someone that they are an addict, oftentimes, they don't want to hear it.

It's said that sugar is more addictive to the brain than cocaine is, so I do realize the challenge when I start messing with your food; it's like messing with a drug addict by trying to take their substance away. When I'm trying to pull sugar away from you, you tend to get testy, start justifying, or flat out reject the information; but I can tell you that it has major consequences if action is not taken.

You may not be familiar with a PET scan, but a PET scan is performed in search of cancer inside the body. Before you do this test, they have you drink a sugary liquid. Attached to the sugar molecule is a radioactive molecule, which they put into the body. Cancer eats the sugar molecule and its attached component. When they radiate you, the imaging lights up the cancer, because the cancer has eaten the radioactive molecule. This proves that most cancers eat what?—sugar.

Now, I know it may not be a hundred percent of cancer cases that act this way, but a good majority of cancer feeds off this toxic substance.

Plus, that spare tire around your waist, that stubborn weight that's been around the thighs and in the face and in the neck, that excess weight that you're carrying around is not fat; it's excess sugar. You put in so much excess energy during the day that your body has to come up with a solution as to what to do with it. So, it stores it away as fat. Thus, if you want to burn fat, you first have to cut sugar.

We don't just want lighter caskets, we want healthier people!

Don't think I'm letting you skinny people off the hook! Not having a weight problem doesn't mean you are healthy. Plenty of skinny people are sick. The same guidelines still apply. If you do not need to lose weight, you still need to cut back sugar and focus on healthy fat and clean protein to keep your weight up.

70% of Americans are overweight yet eat fuel 3-6 times per day. They carry around excess fuel but can't access it, so they need to eat more. They can't get to the fat for fuel, so they keep putting in carbs. It's like a fuel truck that runs out of gas on the side of the road because it can't access what it's carrying. We need to tap into our excess fuel.

Your car runs off of whichever fuel you put into it. If you do not have a car meant for diesel but you fuel it with diesel, then you will have problems. Sugar is like diesel fuel. It burns unclean and leaves a bunch of smoke or damage behind. Fat is like jet fuel and burns much cleaner for your system.

For that reason, we need to reduce the sugar. Don't omit all the carbs, because vegetables are healthy carbs—those are fine. Real-food carbs are great, especially once goals are hit. We just need to get things back in balance. We need to find all the hidden sugars and all the fake-food carbs that turn to sugar and eliminate those. If you want to burn fat, you can't keep fueling with sugar.

- Avoid all bread, crackers, grains, rice, brown rice, chips, oatmeal, cereals, cookies, tortillas, pasta, fried foods, and baked goods—all of these instantly turn to sugar in the body! For now, even if they are real food, they have to go until our body and its reliance on sugar heals.
- Avoid flour and grains. Use almond or coconut flour instead.
- Avoid all soda, sweet tea, alcohol, and sugary drinks—drink regular tea and water.
- Avoid all fruits, fruit drinks, and canned fruits—except granny smith apples, grapefruit, limes, lemons, and moderate amounts of berries. All other fruit instantly turns to high sugar levels in your body.
- Avoid tubers: potatoes, sweet potatoes, and yams, and minimize carrots... they turn to sugar!
- Avoid anything on the ingredients label that has ingredients ending in –ose, i.e., fructose, glucose, maltose, high fructose corn syrup, etc. These are found in mayonnaise, ketchup, yogurt, sodas, and many other packaged goods.
- Avoid all sweeteners including cane juice, brown sugar, syrups, agave nectar, honey, and all artificial sweeteners (Splenda, Sweet'N Low, Equal, etc). Use stevia instead.

Do all of this for just 21 days, or until you hit your goals. Remember that in order to break your sugar addiction, you must get it all out, even healthier sugars like oatmeal and fruit—all sugar must go. When goals are hit, you can add healthy sugar back in, such as fruits, honey, whole grains, potatoes, etc.; but for now, they all have to go.

2. Crank Up the Fat.

You need fat to burn fat! Most of the cells in your body are made of fat. Up to 60% of your brain is made of fat. 39 Healthy fat is essential to your health; bad fat is toxic. The low- and no-fat craze hit America over 40 years ago to combat heart disease. What happened? We got fat! Since then, heart disease has skyrocketed. Fat is not the cause of heart disease, sugar is! All that extra weight around your gut is excess sugar that is stored as fat. Sugar can make good fat/cholesterol turn bad quickly.

If you want to burn up all the fat in your body, one thing must happen nutritionally: you must stop eating sugar. If you do not have sugar as your fuel because you are not eating any of it, then your fuel source becomes fat; you then need to eat fat to spark the engines.

- Avoid rancid fats and oils like margarine, shortening, corn oil, cottonseed oil, vegetable oil, canola oil, soybean oil, safflower oil, and other hydrogenated oils. Use pure olive oil for salads and coconut, avocado or grapeseed oil for all cooking. Also, use organic butter.
- Avoid oil-roasted nuts, seeds, and butter; eat them in their raw or dry roasted form. No oil-roasted, sugar-coated, or flavored nuts and seeds. Cashews, walnuts, almonds, sunflower seeds, flaxseeds, sesame seeds, pine nuts, hemp seeds, macadamias, pecans, and coconut, along with their butter, are great raw options.
- Avoid milk and milk-based products. Use coconut, almond, or cashew milk.
- Increase healthy fats through olives, avocados, nuts, seeds, nut milk, nut butter, clean oils, clean dairy, and clean meats and eggs. (See Protein)

3. Clean Up the Protein.
This is not a high protein/low carb lifestyle change. Protein is very important, but you don't want too much of it because if you overdo it, it will turn to sugar and be hard on your filters (kidneys, liver, etc). Women should eat 15-20 grams per meal, and men should eat 20-30 grams per meal. It is most

important that the protein is "clean." Bioaccumulation of toxins is way higher in a non-organic, hormone-laden, 2,000-pound cow than in a head of broccoli. If finances are a concern and you find it difficult to eat healthily because of the cost, then focus on the proteins. You'll get the most bang for your buck decreasing toxins when you focus on cleaning up meat and dairy products.

You are not what you eat;
you are what you eat, ate.

So, the three main targets for this are beef, chicken, and fish. Pork is out—what does a pig eat? Everything! This makes them very toxic.

A cow is supposed to eat grass. When you feed a cow grain, it grows faster, but the cow becomes inflamed and sick. The cow is then pumped full of growth hormones, which makes for more meat, but it starts to get even sicker, so it must be pumped full of antibiotics. Just before it gets too sick to live, it makes it to market and ends up on your plate.

So, cleaning up the beef that you're eating is crucial. Make sure it's organic and grass-fed when possible to eliminate those hormones, pesticides used in food, and antibiotics.

When it comes to chicken, we're looking for free-range chicken, not a chicken that's cooped up with 10,000 other chickens standing in their own... well, you know what I'm talking about. Oftentimes, they're fed arsenic in order for them to grow quicker. A chicken in today's world is several times larger than a chicken just 50 or 60 years ago because of all the growth hormones and chemicals that are added in to try to make more meat, meaning more profit for the food industry. So, make sure it's organic and free-range when possible to eliminate all those toxic chemicals.

Finally, wild-caught fish: Instead of salmon or tilapia raised on a farm, confined to a pen, and fed pellets and unnatural foods, you want them free in nature. They then consume what they're designed to consume so that toxins don't end up in you, the top of the food chain.

Avoid bottom feeders. Eating these types of animals means you are eating animals that eat everything. They tend to be way more unclean and hold a lot of toxins. The two most common are pork and seafood. What does a pig eat? Anything, so when you eat pork you not only ingest whatever chemicals it ate, but pigs have no sweat glands and tend to hold a lot of toxicity. Shrimp, scallops, clams, and other seafood feed off the bottom and tend to be higher in heavy metals and toxins found in our sea. I'm not saying to never eat them, but at least limit it to special "vacation day" meals.

- Animal Protein – Organic when possible. Grass-fed beef, free-range chicken, and wild-caught fish, as well as grass-fed collagen protein powder. Avoid pork and shellfish.
- Eggs – Free-range, cage-free, organic, and antibiotic- and hormone-free.
- Raw nuts, seeds, and their butter and milk.
- Dairy – Organic milk (but ideally, coconut or almond milk), raw cheese, kefir, full-fat plain yogurt (in moderation).
- No soy products, as they are the number one GMO food on the planet, the second is corn—avoid them both.

So, if you want the most out of decreasing the toxicity in your body, start with cleaning up your proteins first. This also applies to protein in a smoothie. Try to use the grass-fed sourced protein that doesn't have sugar in it and is sweetened with stevia or monk fruit. I avoid whey protein, as it is a source of dairy I can avoid and it spikes insulin levels. Many vegetarian proteins have lots of carbs and tend to spike insulin. For these reasons, I focus more on collagen protein as it supports healthy joints, skin, hair, nails, gut health, and does not spike insulin.

4. Care About Nutrients.

It's amazing to me how many children in this country get very little to no nutrients. From whom do you think they learn that? It's amazing to me how many adults in this country get very little to no nutrients.

Throughout the day, a lot can go wrong when it comes to eating right—eat fast food, don't eat at all, eat late. The easiest and most convenient way to take one step toward fixing your food is through breakfast. I believe we have the most opportunity to add health to our lives through breakfast.

The easiest and most convenient way that I found to really alter breakfast is through a breakfast smoothie or low-carb green juice. In this book, I have included several of my favorite smoothie recipes for you. These are go-to smoothie and juice recipes that I use on a regular basis to get nutrients into my body and to keep toxicity out.

Putting two huge handfuls of spinach or kale or collard greens into your smoothie is a big way to get a huge dose of nutrients for breakfast. I mean, think about it—when was the last time you had a big bowl of spinach for breakfast? Never. Instead, you have a big bowl of oatmeal, which, by the way, turns immediately into sugar because it's a grain. Furthermore, you put brown sugar and craisins on top of it for an extra dose of the insulin spiking toxin.

There are so many other superfoods we could focus on eating rather than oatmeal—we've been sold a lie by Quaker Oats. There are many other things you could do to help your cholesterol, rather than eating a bowl of grain which turns into sugar. Instead, let's get massive amounts of vegetables into your diet in the morning. You will not even taste them when you put them into your smoothie.

In the smoothie, I add lots of veggies like spinach and kale, and then some berries. This keeps the sugar down. Then, I add good fat like coconut milk, almond milk, or coconut oil. Next, a scoop of my greens powder supercharges the drinks with 50+ nutrients and 15 extra servings of fruits and veggies. Finally, I get protein by adding my grass-fed collagen protein powder, which doubles as a multivitamin as well. This hits the first four C's, fills me up, energizes me, and gets a majority of my nutrients first thing in the morning. Make one as big as you would like!

Some days I just do the greens powder or buy a really low carbohydrate green juice and add my greens powder to it for a very fast and convenient, supercharged breakfast. During the rest of the day, I focus on getting more nutrients by adding vegetables to each meal, taking greens powder, opting for salads, eating beans—sautéed, baked, or steamed, or dipping my favorite veggies in hummus or guac.

Fuel your vehicle, not your cravings.

From a beverage standpoint, you're just going to focus

on water, the essential nutrient. Up to 70% of your body is made of water, so pour the water in, enjoy it, add a lemon or cucumber to it, and put good water inside your system. I also like to add in my greens powder and my energizing vitamin c powder to help absorb the water better. Tea and coffee are okay; however, alcohol should be avoided. Just make sure you don't fill your coffee and tea with toxins or sugars.

As for nutrient-dense snacks, here are some ideas:
- Veggies (peppers, cucumbers, broccoli, etc.) with hummus
- A boiled egg with salt and pepper
- Avocado with salt and pepper
- Handfuls of raw nuts
- A granny smith apple with almond butter
- A tea or small coffee with some organic cream, coconut milk, almond milk, and/or stevia
- A blended coffee with butter, coconut oil, and Collagen Protein (Bulletproof Coffee)

You have got to find ways throughout the day to get greens into your system, just like the spinach in the smoothie. If you constantly put nutrients in, your body is going to have the raw materials to work well. The food isn't the healer, it's the doctor on the inside that gets the good stuff to work with that brings the healing.

The reason that superfoods, oils, or supplements work so well is that they're actually nutritious raw materials that the body can actually do something with. If you give the body rotten, unstable material to build the building, the building is going to crumble very easily and collapse. If you give it strong, fortified nutrients and raw materials to work with, you're going to have a strong foundation.

So, you have to care about the nutrients you eat. You're not eating to satisfy your taste buds; you're eating to be healthy and build a strong foundation.

5. Curb Your Consumption.

If you are struggling to still lose weight and hit health goals after the above four C's of nutrition, then curb your consumption. Take a fasting approach. Fasting is an ancient technique that just may be exactly what overconsuming America needs.

Don't let the word scare you. There are several techniques that are incredibly effective at lowering your insulin which puts you in fat-burning mode. The longer you are in that state the more you will burn. Fasting has a huge impact on your system and health.

Some of us have not gone a single day of our life without eating. Think about that! When you take a few meals or days off from eating, you are finally giving your digestive tract a day off after years of 7-days-a-week work. All that extra energy your body conserves can now be used to HEAL you. Fasting prolongs life, lowers inflammation, and enhances detoxification.[45] I use it weekly. There are three ways I do this:

1. Do the old "Slim-Fast Method." Eat a smoothie for breakfast, a smoothie for lunch, and then a sensible dinner (Note: Skip using Slim Fast or any other pre-made shake— they are toxic and loaded with sugars!) Although not true fasting it is curbing consumption and a great place to start.
2. Intermittent Fasting. Only eat food from 12:00 p.m. – 6:00 p.m. or any six-hour window. Have lunch and dinner, and then give your body a chance to spend all its energy on healing you for the next 18 hours.
3. Rotational Fasting. This is the most powerful technique I

have seen when it comes to resetting your metabolism. How long has it taken you to put on weight and be addicted and dependent on so much food? Years! So if our systems have been slowly damaged, then they need to be nurtured and slowly repaired.

Have you ever started a workout regime or diet and got really good results for a few weeks and then plateaued? If yes, then your body figured out how to adjust to the new normal regimen. To break through this plateau with exercise you change the intensity, timing, and length of exercise and your body again changes. The same applies to your metabolism, it needs to be challenged with different frequency, size, and timing of meals so it does not plateau.

In your workbook, you will find an advanced meal plan that will give you a slight change each week to challenge your body differently to avoid plateauing and keep progressing. Most do not need to jump to this first, but it is another tool I deploy regularly to keep my body healing and progressing.

You will be hungry, but you will also realize we MASSIVELY overeat in America! You'll live! We need to re-establish our relationship with food. Embrace that hunger pain. That's just you resetting the outrageous consumption habit you developed. Over time your body will adjust, and you'll be shocked how you are actually NOT hungry; it was just a bad habit.

Keep in mind that as you go through this plan, it is quite a shock to the system in the first couple of days. When you're used to having four coffees a day, when you're used to having alcohol, when you're used to having lots and lots of sugar, when you're used to having Starbucks Frappuccinos, when you're used to drinking and eating processed food by man, it's a shock to the system to take it away.

So, at first, you may be headachy and/or nauseated, your energy may change, and/or your digestion may change. But once you get over the three-to-seven-day hump, you'll really start to level out; your energy will start going up and you'll see the weight coming off. You'll see the blood pressure leveling, the blood sugar coming down, and some massive changes, along with healing, as you fix your food.

If you owned a Lamborghini, you wouldn't put poor-quality fuel in it; you would put in the highest-quality fuel possible, to make it perform the way it's designed to perform. That's what you are—you're a Lamborghini. You may not feel like one, but the performance that your body is capable of is out-of-this-world powerful. It's actually quite impressive how well it still performs, despite your loading it up with sugar, junk food, drugs, and toxins. Imagine what's possible with no toxins! Give yourself clean rocket fuel and watch yourself go. Pour a bunch of water on top of that, and you're going to be feeling amazing.

—————————— BONUS "C" ——————————

Consider Supplements.

In today's world, I do not see supplements as a recommendation, but a requirement. If all you did was implement the lifestyle change in this book, you'd get amazing results, but supplements surely make up for deficiencies and make things easier.

Our food and soil are losing their nutrient supply. Unless you are eating all of your food straight out of your own nutrient-dense soil in your garden, then chances are you are not getting the nutrients you need. When comparing the content of 13 different nutrients found in 43 crops, scientists found that on average, the soil content has declined 6% to 38% for different nutrients in our soil over the last 100 years. You have to eat more fruits and veggies to get the nutrients you need. So supplementation is not Just a recommendation—it is a requirement.[46]

Supplements still need to follow the same rules as real food. Many people make this mistake. All-day long, I analyze supplements for patients, and I consistently see the same mistakes. After 25,000+ patients, here are the most common supplement mistakes:

- Cut the Sugar. Just like in food, rule number one is often violated. Especially powdered supplements, but pill form, too. Watch out for whey proteins, corn, maltodextrin, and any form of fructose or sugar names we have discussed.
- Crank Up the Good Fat. This also means removing the bad fat. Poor quality supplements are loaded with soybean oils and rancid fish oils.
- Clean up the Toxins. As discussed with food, supplements have some common toxins. Here are the most common I see:
  » Magnesium Stearate (Vegetable Stearate is ok)
  » Toxic Dyes (Red 40, Blue 2, etc)
  » Titanium Dioxide
  » Soy
  » Whey Protein From Non-Grass-Fed Cows
  » Whey Isolate (Highly Processed and Contains Heavy Metals)
- Care About Nutrients. Supplement ingredients made from real foods with no gluten, wheat, dairy, or genetically-modified foods are crucial. Just like with the guidelines of

food, we want high-quality, real ingredients in supplements.

- Vitamin D. Vitamin D2 is synthetic vitamin D that is often prescribed. D3 is a healthy form. Every 1000 IU of vitamin D must be taken with 100 mg of vitamin k to prevent calcification of the arteries. K1 and 2 forms of K2 are ideal (MK-4 and MK-7). Your body uses magnesium to convert vitamin D in your body, so magnesium should also be taken to ensure absorption and avoid magnesium deficiencies. Vitamin D is fat-soluble and should be taken with a healthy fat for better absorption, as well as the other fat-soluble vitamins A, E, and K so they can work synergistically.

- Omegas. These should be sourced from freshwater fish and in the naturally-occurring triglyceride form. To protect the quality, it should be in non-transparent containers with less than 120 capsules. Watch out for toxic additives, colorings, and bad fats. A high dose of Omega 3s to cut down inflammation and healthy Omega 6, 7, and 9s are a plus. Antioxidants should be added to protect the oil's quality.

- Multi-Vitamins. Avoid toxic additives, colorings, and sugars. If they contain B vitamins, be sure they are the methyl forms, to avoid sensitivity issues to non-methylated forms. An example would be to take folic acid in the folate form.

- Greens. Make sure the greens powder contains no sugars, or forms of sugar ending in -ose, maltodextrin, or the toxic additives above. Ideally, it should be dairy-, GMO-, and wheat-free. Make sure they are 3rd-party tested for heavy metals and pesticides. Ideally, keep it as organic as possible with a wide range of fruits, veggies, and nutrients.

- Collagen. Collagen does not spike insulin levels like other protein powders. Collagen depletes with age, so it is needed to support the skin, hair, and nails, and to repair the gut and joints. Be sure it is sourced from grass-fed, free-range animals. Be sure there are no added sugars.

Mine also contains my multivitamins to consolidate.

- Probiotics. Make sure they do not contain fillers and toxins. They must be in a stable form so they don't spoil, or are killed before they get deep into your gut. You can get most of these by eating raw vegetables and fermented food like sauerkraut, kombucha, kefir, and apple cider vinegar. I get mine through foods and the greens powder.
- Calcium. Most people do not need calcium supplementation; they need mineral balance. Science suggests to not take more than 600mg per day, especially if you have heart and blood vessel issues. For bone strength, it has to be taken with magnesium, vitamin D, and vitamin K.
- Other supplements to consider are vitamin C, turmeric, zinc, and magnesium.

This can all be much easier than it sounds. Everyone always asks, "What does Dr. Livingood do?" or "What do you take, Doc?" Well, each day I start my day with greens that contain a huge nutrient dose, probiotics, digestive enzymes, and can be added to my morning juice/smoothie. I then take my collagen protein which gives me clean protein and my multivitamins including B vitamins, magnesium, and zinc. I put that right in my organic coffee with healthy fats (bulletproof coffee). I take my vitamin D complex with A, E, K, zinc, and magnesium included for my immune system, as well as my complete omega, so that the healthy oils help absorb the vitamin D. Later in the day, I have some vitamin C powder to support my adrenals, electrolytes, and brain and heart helpers to keep me energized and focused in the afternoons.

Five supplements get me all my nutrients and replace a meal each day for me, so it saves me a ton of time and money. Three easy-to-use, delicious powders that replace breakfast and afternoon cravings, and two other pill-form supplements—

that's it. If I need a snack before I get home for a healthy dinner, I eat raw nuts, veggies, and hummus, or a nutrient-filled Livingood Daily Bar. During the workweek this keeps me light, filled with nutrients, and able to enjoy vacation meals on the weekends.

Take little steps. Develop habits and start replacing bad foods and supplements. Just changing your thinking and fixing your food will bring massive transformation, but there are more layers to go in this health onion! Let's go deeper.

NECK SURGERY HAS BEEN CANCELED! OFF STOMACH AND PAIN MEDS!

VERTIGO, DIZZINESS, FATIGUE, DEPRESSION, AND ANXIETY ALL GONE!

OFF 3 MEDICATION, REFLUX IS GONE, SLEEPING BETTER, AND NO MORE ALLERGY AND SINUS ISSUES!

7

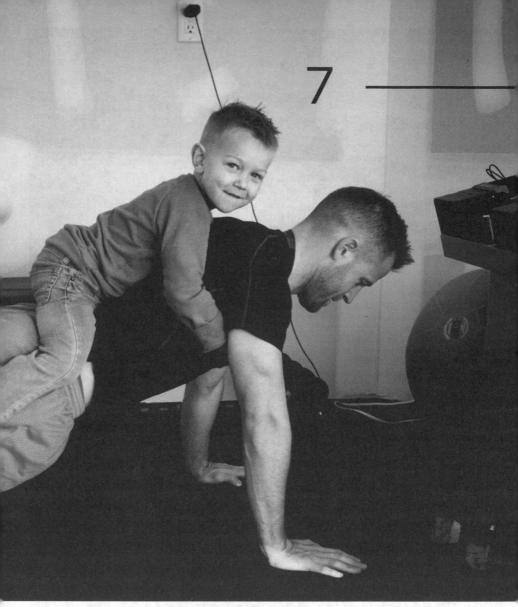

Whenever I feel the need to exercise I
lie down until it goes away."
– Paul Terry

"Those who think they have no time for
bodily exercise will sooner or later have
to find time for illness."
– Edward Stanley

CHAPTER SEVEN

FIX YOUR FITNESS

Oxygen is extremely important for the body. Too much carbon dioxide buildup in the body is not good, and not enough oxygen deep in the tissues causes the body to become toxic. If you don't believe it, go ahead and hold your breath—see how long you'll last. Oxygen is required to run every function inside of our body; however, most diseases can't survive in highly oxygenated environments.

So, how do you get oxygen in? The simplest, most efficient way to kill disease, lose weight, and experience real health is movement. But, how you move makes all the difference.

If there were a way to actually get into shape in 10 minutes a day, with no gym, with no equipment, with no cost—would you like to know how to do that?

Now, this goes against the old approach to exercise. Spending hours in the gym, running or walking for hours on treadmills, or running for long distances can be fulfilling for some. I mix up workouts occasionally, or even do 5K's myself for fun with my family. But when it comes to the optimal function of your body, it's all about short bursts, more muscle, less fat, less sugar in your system, and optimized hormones.

A typical long-distance runner's body will have fat stored in reserve for long runs. Instead of bulky sprinter muscles, a long-distance runner will have smaller, more slender muscles. A person doing higher intensity, shorter durations like a sprinter, is going to have higher amounts of muscle mass. The more muscle a person has, the higher their fat burning will be. They'll burn sugar quickly, melt away fat, and be much more toned.

Most people I come across want to be more toned up, they want more muscle, they want more physique, and they want to drop the fat. The best way to do that is high-intensity, short-duration workouts. Work out like a sprinter, not a marathoner... it's all about hormones.

Hormones inside of your body are the key to unlocking weight loss and fitness.

Too much or too little of specific hormones can quickly alter your fitness. For example, testosterone—when you do high-intensity, short-duration workouts, you get up to a 771% testosterone boost, more than any other type of workout. The more testosterone a person has, the more muscle is built and the less fat there is.[40]

Consider hormones like cortisol, the stress hormone. Do you need more stress hormones in your life? Longer distance and longer workouts create more stress on our bodies.[41] Short duration, high-intensity workouts decrease cortisol, giving you a sense of relief; it also increases your dopamine and serotonin hormones and makes you happier.

Insulin might be the biggest bully hormone you have. It suppresses good hormones and enhances the wrong ones, like stress. When you do high-intensity, short-duration workouts, you're burning up the sugar that's in your blood. Once you burn up all the sugar in your body, your body is now out of that fuel and has to switch to its other fuel, which is fat. That starts to reset the insulin receptors in your body; it starts allowing you to be a fat-burner, instead of a sugar-burner. It suppresses insulin, and your body loves it. If you don't eat sugar and just eat fat, you will supercharge this type of workout to burn fat! Hormones allow your body to burn more fat instead of storing fat. High-intensity, short-duration workouts are more the way I believe our bodies were designed to work. As amazing as they are, we can still do longer duration workouts. We can still do runs, walks, triathlons, and Ironmans. But if you're looking for quick, time-saving results, high-intensity, short-duration workouts are the key.

10 Minute Workout

High-intensity workouts can be simple. These workouts use your own body weight so you don't need a gym or equipment, and anyone can do them, whether you are a Level 1 Beginner, Level 2 Advanced, or somewhere in between.

1. Pick three exercises. (push-ups, jumping jacks, squats, lunges, running in place, or side-to-side jumps, for example.)
2. Do the first exercise for 50 seconds as fast as you can. Intensity is the key.
3. Take a 10-second break.
4. Do the second exercise for 50 seconds as fast as you can. Intensity is the key.
5. Take another 10-second break.
6. Do the third exercise for 50 seconds as fast as you can. Intensity is the key.
7. Take a 40-second break, that's the end of round 1.
8. Repeat this routine for two more rounds.

Nine minutes and 50 seconds, that's it! Get on with your day and feel good about yourself!

You are 10 minutes-a-day to a new you! There are two keys to results, though. The first key is intensity. That means you want your heart rate at 70% plus of your maximum heart rate; you want to be breathing heavily and working hard. If you're not breathing heavily and can talk to your neighbor, you're not doing it hard enough.

You have to breathe hard to burn fat.

Key number two is consistency. You can't do just 10 minutes of exercise once a week!

Do the 10 Minute Workout six days a week— that's ONE HOUR of exercise per week— and you can get yourself into shape!

Switch up the exercises and incorporate weights or equipment, if you'd like to mix it up. The beauty is that this can be done anywhere with no equipment, in a short amount of time. Bye-bye excuses! Just do it!

Research shows once you are done with the high-intensity workout in which you surged your fat-burning hormones, your hormones will keep surging over the next 14-24 hours. You'll burn more fat using a 10-minute workout than if you did a moderate-intensity workout for an hour in the gym.[42]

Go as hard as you can, surge your hormones, surge your body's ability to burn fat, then rest—and do it again. Short bursts of energy are going to maximize and fire-up the fat-burning machine inside of you.

My wife and I do these together several times a week. With her first pregnancy, she gained 50 pounds. During her second pregnancy, she did the 10-Minute Workout every day (including the day she had our little girl, London!) and only gained 25 pounds! If a 9-month pregnant momma can do this, what's your excuse?

As part of our challenges, we give people on-demand, press-play, follow-along workouts to make it even easier. You don't have to come up with the workout; you can just follow along with us as we encourage you and guide you through. This is also a perfect time to throw in a 2-minute ab bonus and stretching to help fix your frame. We'll talk more about that soon.

When you think differently, start fixing your food, and implement this type of workout, you'll see quick changes. You are still only halfway to experiencing real health. Do not make the mistake my dad made and miss the last *T* of interference; keep the right goals in mind.

AMANDA COULDN'T GET PREGNANT AND NOW IS! NOT TO MENTION DAD'S HEADACHES, NECK PAIN AND NUMBNESS/TINGLING ARE GONE!

IN JUST 2 MONTHS, CHUCK IS OFF OF 5 PAIN MEDICATIONS!

IMPROVED AUTOIMMUNE DISORDER AND OFF 6 MEDICATIONS!

8 ——————

"The master of your body did not run off and leave you masterless."
– BJ Palmer

"Look well to the spine for the cause of disease."
– Hippocrates

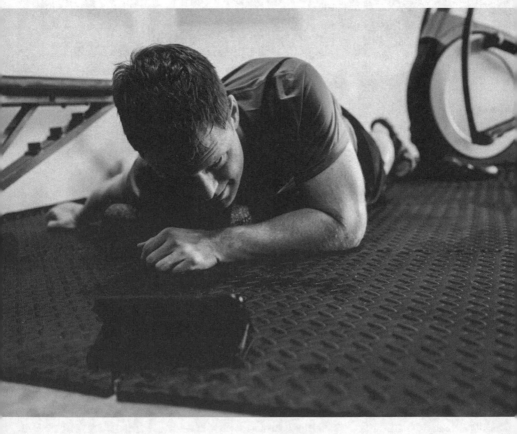

CHAPTER EIGHT
FIX YOUR FRAME

You can get nutrition right. You can get fitness right. You can get stress right. You can get supplements right. But if you miss the last *T*, it can be devastating to your health. The third *T* of the causes of interference is Trauma.

What is the most important organ you have? If you said your heart, what controls your heart? It's your brain. God put an amazing healing power in your brain; it sends messages down your spinal cord and across your nerves to every organ, cell, and tissue inside your body. It beats your heart, it breathes your lungs, and it tells you how to love someone. For you to be reading this book right now, your brain has to tell your body how to do that.

If I take a pair of scissors and cut the nerve going to your heart, what happens to your heart? It stops. It's dead.

If I pinch or damage the nerve coming out of the lower part of your neck that's controlling the beating of your heart, does your heart get healthier or does it get sicker? It gets sicker.

If I leave that damage in there a day, a month, a year, five years, ten years—what will eventually happen to your heart? It's going to stop.

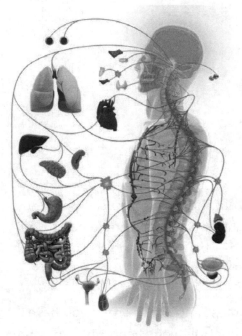

If there's damage on the nerve going to your heart and I give your heart drugs, does that fix the problem? Absolutely not.

If there's damage on a nerve going to your heart and I take the old one out and put a new one in, does that fix the problem? No. If I give you the best nutrition on the planet, does that fix the problem? No. If I give you a supplement, does that fix the problem? No. If you exercise every day, does that fix the problem? No.

The problem lies in the blockage of the nerve getting the healing from the brain to your heart. Until that pressure is removed, the body can't heal 100%. I'm not saying that exercise and nutrition wouldn't be a good thing, but before you can do those things, you must get the inside healing and working at 100%, or as close to 100% as possible. That key lies in taking care of your nervous system.

That's what happened to my dad. He had four car accidents before he was 18 years of age. In his thirties, he fell out of a tree onto his head. He sat driving a truck all day. He damaged his nervous system at a very young age and, by the time he got to age 51, his heart hit that 60% functioning threshold. That's when his symptoms first showed up in the form of his heart shutting down. It was all because he had damage on a nerve going to his heart, and he had no idea it was there.

Could you have an artery blocked and not know it? Absolutely. Could you have a nerve blocked and not know it? Absolutely.

Your frame's job is to hold you up against gravity and protect you from trauma. Your spine is one of the most important pieces as it surrounds and protects your nervous system and holds your posture upright. The nervous system is completely surrounded by bone to protect the most delicate system you have. When you look at your spine, it must be nice and straight from the front with your hips level. From the side, it has to have three 35-45 degree curves. The strongest structure known to man is the arch, and you have three of them in your spine to hold you up and protect your nervous system. Brilliant design!

Simply put, there are three main parts to your nervous system, and these must be fully intact to experience real health. Here they are:

Part 1 is your brain stem. Your brainstem controls all the subconscious functions of your body; it tells your blood pressure how to go up and down, it controls your blood sugar, and it controls the acid in your stomach. Your sleep, your mood, and your concentration are all controlled by your brainstem.

Right, where your brain stem comes out of the base of your skull is actually called the *Foramen Magnum* or "Mouth of God"; that "Mouth of God" is where the brainstem connects your brain and your spinal cord, which is the power source to the rest of your body. That area is surrounded and protected by a bone called the atlas. Do you remember the Greek figure of the man holding the world on his back? His name was Atlas. The top bone of the spine is named the same because it holds up your world!

A famous person who has damaged this bone is Christopher Reeve; you may remember him as Superman back in the 1980s. Christopher Reeve was riding along on a horse, fell off, and jammed his chin into the ground. He damaged his atlas, the first bone of his neck. In fact, it moved over a quarter of an inch into his brainstem and shut that area down immediately.

Christopher Reeve damaged one bone in his neck, and what happened to his legs? He couldn't move his legs, he needed a pacemaker for his heart, and he needed a respirator tube for his lungs. Someone had to push on his belly just so he could go to the bathroom.

Christopher Reeve did not have bad organs! He had a bad what?—connection—a bad nervous system and spine. So many people are treating organs instead of first looking at the thing controlling them, the nervous system. Can you see how important that little bone called the atlas and your brainstem are to your overall health? If you ask Christopher Reeve, it's everything.

The first place to start when it comes to true health care is right at the top.

ADIO (Above-down, inside-out).

The power inside your body works from your brain, down through your spinal cord, and out through the nerves to the organs in your body. Oftentimes, we'll get stuck on treating the organ—outside-in, below-up. We really need to get to the cause—what's controlling it—the nervous system.

Part two of your nervous system is your spinal cord. How important is your spinal cord? If you damage it, you're paralyzed. Your spinal cord is a river of life flowing down through your spine to carry all the messages and all the healing everywhere in your body. This river of life must be protected by the three properly-functioning curves mentioned above. There's a curve in your neck, another one in your mid-back, and one in your lower back.

"Sitting is the new smoking."

Part number two is hindered by sitting—"the new smoking." It's said that you can smoke a cigarette, and it will take 11 minutes off of your life; but if you sit sedentarily, watching TV for one hour, it can take up to 22 minutes off of your life. Now, if you sit watching TV for one hour, while smoking cigarettes, I don't even know the math on that; but, as a doctor, I would highly not recommend it.

"Sitting is the new smoking" because of the damage it does to your spinal cord. There have to be three distinct curves in your spine; when there is, your spinal cord is protected.

Think of a banana (the next time you eat a banana, you'll think of me). When you have a curved banana, the peel protects the pulp. When you straighten a banana, what do you have? You've got a mashed banana. That same thing happens to your spinal cord when you lose the curve in your neck. Make a C with your hand right now. If you feel your palm, it feels nice and soft. If you straighten your hand, just like straightening a banana, you feel your skin stretching, along with the muscles that control that area. That's exactly what happens and exactly what it looks like when you stretch and lose the curvature in your spine.

This is what makes sitting the new smoking. When you lose the curvature in your neck, it's been tied to decreased breathing rates, decreased heart function, and an increase in allergies and asthma.[31]

Loss of spinal curves has been shown to increase mortality and take up to 14 years off of your life.[32]

When you lose the curves, it creates a horrible posture and puts incredible strain on your nervous system.

In fact, for every inch that your head moves forward in front of your shoulders, you have an extra ten pounds of weight that will be carried on the bottom of your neck on that spinal cord and the nerves. They call this the posture of looking at your own grave.[33]

What do we do most of the day? Sit. We sit in front of computers, we sit in front of the TV, and we sit while we drive. Texting neck - looking down at your cell phone or completely straight down to the floor puts an extra 60 pounds of pressure on your neck![34] We sleep in weird positions and we sit in weird positions on the couch. Let alone if you've been in a car accident, had some kind of injury/trauma, or participated in athletic events, you've definitely damaged this arch of life, which is the cervical curve in your neck.

If any of the three curves are lost inside of your body, scientific studies have proven that it directly correlates to dysfunction and disease in your organs, and herein lies the cause of most diseases we now see. The reason you get disease in one area, or in one organ but not another is due to the damage to the nerve controlling that organ.

Daily posture exercises and caring for your frame is a must in today's technological world.

Part 3 of your nervous system is the nerves. The brainstem connects itself to the brain. The brainstem then connects to the spinal cord, and then the messages that the spinal cord carries are sent out into the body through the nerves like telephone wires.

Your spine, from the front, protects those nerves. From the front, your spine must be nice and straight, and your hips must be level. As long as it's straight, there's no damage to the nervous system, and the messages can get from there into the body uninterrupted—you're healthy.

I'm sure you've heard of the condition scoliosis. Scoliosis is a significant curvature in the spine, which is supposed to be straight. When you see a 40 or 50 or 80-degree scoliosis that looks like a snake, what does the doctor recommend that person do right away? Surgery with two big rods to try to straighten the spine. Why would they do that? Studies have proven that bad scoliosis in a person's spine takes 14 years off of their life because it damages the nervous system and shuts down the organs that are on the other end.[35]

If 60-degree scoliosis causes early death for someone, what about 40 degrees or 20 degrees, or even two degrees? What if there are right now two degrees of pressure on the nerve that goes to your heart? What if there are two degrees of pressure on the nerve that goes to your child's heart? What if there are two degrees of pressure on the nerve going into your wife's reproductive system? What if there are two degrees of damage to the brainstem of your father or your mother? Are you concerned?

Now, let me ask you this. What if there are no symptoms, and you have one degree of damage or two degrees of damage, or 20 degrees of damage? If you sent a person to a medical doctor today and they didn't have any symptoms, but their spine had shifted, what would the doctor say? They're fine.

In fact, we don't even have a name for it until it reaches 10 degrees; then we call it scoliosis. If the curve is 20-40 degrees, they'll do bracing or therapies; if the curve goes above 40 degrees and they are old enough, medical doctors will do surgery... a $150,000 Harrington Rod surgery.

My point here is that even a medical doctor knows that a bad back, a bad neck, or a bad spine causes sickness, disease, and early death; they just don't know what to do, nor are they trained to do anything about it until it's a crisis.

Do you want to wait until you or your family is in a crisis to take care of a problem? That's what we've been trained to do in America. As soon as there's a crisis, we'll start addressing it. We've got to start taking care of our frame now.

2 Fixing-Your-Frame Tips

1. Fix Your Sit.

Sitting 8+ hours per day is horrible for your joints, organs, and weight. You have to find a way to stand more. Get a standing desk, set a timer to take walk breaks, or stretch breaks. If you do sit, then I would advise lumbar support, which is a simple roll that straps onto your chair to put the curve into your lower back so you do not slouch. Raise your computer screen, lower your chair, or again...stand more.

2. Fix Your Sleep.

Sleeping on your stomach, on your shoulder, or twisted in some weird position causes micro-trauma to your frame. At a minimum, try starting on your back and put a roll/support under your neck and one under your low back to restore the spine's normal curves. Be sure it is no bigger than 3" in diameter for your neck, and 2.5" in diameter for your lower back so you do not overdo it. This is like wearing retainers at night. It gets your frame back to its normal position at least for a few hours. If you do go to your side, support (but do not over-support) your head so your neck isn't tilted. Also, try not to be in a twisted position.

3. BONUS

Upon waking, spend 2 minutes stretching your frame after your 10-minute workout. In our community, we have resources to show you how to do it, as well as individual rehab videos for any joint in your body that you are struggling with. Visit *www. livingooddaily.com* to learn more.

My dad had a bad frame. At the bottom of his neck, he had bad joints that went undetected for many years. If you look at his X-ray, you can see decaying of the spine at the bottom of his neck because of those accidents when he was 16, 17, and 18, because of the falls in his 30's, and because he drove a truck for UPS for 35 years, bouncing up and down. My dad lost the curvature in his neck. Those "tires,"—his spine and discs, stayed out of alignment long enough to wear down. The curves stayed out of alignment long enough that his spine wore down and degenerated the lower part of his neck.

Research shows that when the spine degenerates, the nervous system degenerates.[37] When your spine and nervous system are degenerating, what does it do to your organs on the other end? They shut down as well.

My dad had phase-two degeneration in the lower part of his neck, and it electrically shorted-out his heart at age 51. The same diagnosis was confirmed by Mayo Clinic a few years prior when they put a pacemaker in his heart. They were correct; my dad had an electrical issue with his heart. They just put all their focus and all the treatment where?—on treating the heart and treating the symptoms—no one ever checked the wires. The bottom of my dad's neck held the answer. We had to fix his frame.

We had one of the causes to fix, but we had to battle all the treatment he had done up to this point. Two years of dozens of medications took its toll on my dad. His liver, kidneys, and gut needed help! Some of us have been so off-track for so long that we need to go back and clear out a lot of the damage we have already created, as well as doing better moving forward. We had to undo Dad's previous damage by fixing his filters.

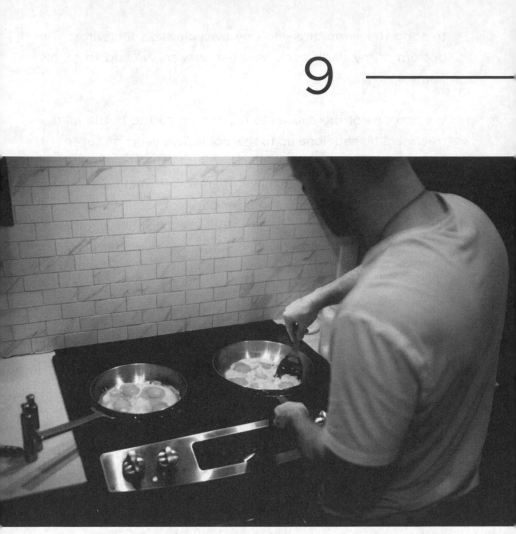

"The doctor of the future will give no medication, but will interest his patients in the care of the human frame, diet, and in the cause and prevention of disease."
– Thomas Edison

CHAPTER NINE
FIX YOUR FILTERS

Are you toxic? Would you like to take a toxicity test? Toxins have an affinity for the eyes, so let's do a simple visual acuity test. Can you read the two exact middle letters in this sentence?

QEFUONRFJJBWDJN

Research shows that if you could see the letters RF, and if you currently live in America and are holding this book, then you are toxic! HAHA! Got ya! But in all seriousness, no expensive toxicity test is needed to know that!

It's impossible to avoid all toxins. One approach is to minimize your exposure to toxins; the second is to rid your body of those already in you. We already dug into the main two causes of toxicity: your food and fitness, but that does not address the many other environmental toxins that affect us.

I do have to stress this again. There is a 99.9% chance you are still WAY off of truly eating real food, eliminating food toxins, and moving your body enough. Want to detox? Then follow and understand the 5 "C" guidelines to nutrition and commit to 10-minute workouts, 6 days a week. When you clean up the nutrients in your body, you're 70% of the way towards eliminating the toxic sources you and your family take in on a daily basis.

When you exercise, you are extracellularly flushing those toxins out of your skin by sweating. You speed up your digestive system, and you're breathing and getting the toxins out. You're amplifying the detox systems when you work out. Many want to blow by this for the "fancier" tips, but simple, consistent changes in nutrition and fitness are some of the best detoxes you can do.

We do, however, live in a toxic environment. The more man interferes with the earth and our bodies, the more toxins we're exposed to. Toxins are impossible to ignore and avoid in today's world.

In this chapter, I'm going to give you the five main steps to follow in order to combat environmental toxins. There are certainly many additional levels to truly deal with challenging toxicity problems, but this chapter will give you and your family the next steps to be implemented on a regular basis.

We ingest four billion prescription drugs in the United States each year. 70,000 chemicals are used commercially. Over 3,000 chemicals are added to our food supply, and over 10,000 chemicals are used in food processing, preserving, and storage.

What can you do then? The principle of detoxifying is this: when you ingest a toxin, your body has got to get it out of you. So, if you were to drink a cup of gasoline, what would your body do? It would throw up—thank God, it got the toxin out of your system. My point is, sometimes when you experience symptoms like throwing-up, diarrhea, or sinus drainage, it's not a bad thing; it's your body getting rid of the bad that's inside of it. If the bad stayed in your body, then that would not be good.

For example, is a fever good or bad? A fever is a great thing! I know, I know, I'm not a fan of 104-degree temperatures, being lethargic, and sweating. I know it may not feel good, but think about it—your body literally knows how to heat up a couple of degrees to get a bacteria or virus out of it. It knows how to sterilize itself. Most of the time, all you're taught to do is take a drug to lower the fever. If your body is trying to sterilize itself to stay well, then that's the last thing you'd want to do.

Diarrhea. It's not fun, but it's a necessary thing. If a toxin gets inside of your body, your system will flush it out. Oftentimes, you need to honor the symptoms you have, knowing it's your body's way of eliminating the toxin that you came in contact with. Of course, be safe; but we would be way better off if more times than not, we just let the body do its thing. After all, it is much smarter than we are!

There are many products out there that detox. I want to focus on five action and prevention steps you can do on a daily basis

108

with your family to focus on diminishing your toxin load. These are simple—I could list 50, but make sure to do these first. Also, I'll briefly touch on how to flush more toxins out of your system by optimizing your "filters" or the detox organs already present in your body.

Here are your top five toxin tips:

1. Avoid Medications

ALL forms of medication are toxic; they are drugs. Remember what would happen to the fish? The average drug comes with 70 different side effects.[26] The fewer drugs you are on, the less toxic you will be, and the healthier you will be. The more you get to the cause of the issue, the fewer drugs you'll ever need to take.

America takes 75% of the world's drugs, yet we make up only 5% of the world's population.[27] We are not healthier because of it; no drug can ever heal you. By the law of human nature, you cannot take a toxin and get healthier. If I give a drug to a dead person, nothing happens. The only thing that can heal you is the power inside of you.

A drug never improves that healing power; it can only interfere with it. Drugs may save someone's life in a crisis—thank God they do that—but they're not designed to make you healthier. If you are on drugs, you should always be actively working toward safely coming off those drugs with the medical provider that put you on them. Medications are our number one toxin. To combat this, follow our wellness cabinet guidelines for powerful, non-toxic alternatives to OTC drugs. Visit *www.livingooddaily.com* for more info.

2. Microbes

Bacteria, viruses, candida, and invaders are absolutely pandemic in the world. I'm not just referring to the flu or coronavirus, but a ton more that cannot be seen or are rarely talked about. Arguably, we are being bombarded with microbes now more than any other time in history. With the number of medical advancements, how are we so plagued with Epstein Barr, corona, and herpes viruses? Nearly every American has those in their system. How many people are housing harmful bacteria and yeast (candida) overgrowth in their guts? How many other foreign invaders are we carrying that we are unaware of?

Every invader needs a good host to survive, and I believe we have made ourselves into a perfect host environment. Continuously weakening our defense system. Taking too many drugs and injections that suppress our immune system Downing entirely too much sugar and bread/carbs have fed many of our guts with yeast overgrowth. The linings of our digestive tracts have an overgrowth of bad bacteria because of our antibiotic overuse. Every harsh treatment and toxic food has a side effect.

For example, dropping an antibiotic bomb on an infection will rid the body of that bacteria, but it will also wipe out the bacteria or "good soldiers" that are actually protecting our systems. Without these good foot soldiers, invaders are able to rise up and take over.

We need more balance. One must begin eating properly in order to stop promoting the systemic imbalance, but here are a few more things to focus on each day to support a healthy gut and strengthen your internal army.

- Take a small dose of probiotics daily. These are the good bacteria to build back up. Fermented foods and raw vegetables are equally a great choice to get these probiotics in via food.
- Combat yeast and candida overgrowth by following the challenge food guidelines. You may also consider a candida cleanse.
- Bolster your defense against viruses by taking coconut oil daily, which is high in lauric acid—a good defender of viruses. Spirulina, chlorella, and lots of greens help the liver detox and deal with viral loads.
- Take ample amounts of vitamin D and fat-soluble vitamins daily, as they help to boost the immune system. Vitamin C, quercetin, and zinc have also been shown to strengthen the immune response.
- Consider colloidal silver, oil of oregano, apple cider vinegar, and/or coconut oil as powerful antifungal, antimicrobial, and antiviral agents for various bodily infections or conditions.

Every day your immune system, which is controlled by your gut, liver, and other filters, gets weaker or stronger. Which way is yours going today? Be proactive toward these toxins, instead of reactive.

See your supplement overview in the "Fix Your Food" chapter, or in the appendix at the back of the book for supplements that facilitate the ingestion of the above listed products and to see how I do it daily for myself and my family.

3. Water

Good, clean, healthy water is so important because, as we said, almost 70% of your body is made of it. So many poor countries of the world don't have clean water. However, many toxins in America come from our water supply. As discussed earlier, it's a disease of excess.

All the chemicals we use end up in our water, and if we don't have filtration systems in place to purify the water, we drink all the harmful toxins. Prescription drugs, fertilizers, hormones, pesticides, and other chemicals are not eliminated from tap water and therefore end up in your body if you aren't careful.

―――――――――――― *Use a filter or be a filter.* ――――――――――――

Purifying your water is a necessity to prevent many of these toxins from entering your body. Clean water also aids your body's detox process. At a minimum, you have to have some sort of filtration in your fridge and faucet. It would also be ideal to have a whole-house filtration system or a reverse osmosis filter somewhere in your house. The only issue with RO is that it removes the minerals, so be sure to add those back in. Filtered bottled water eliminates toxins, but as you'll find out in tip four, the plastics come with other harms. Surface area filtration is your best bet.

You also get a lot of water toxicity from your shower. Gallons and gallons of water pour over you in the shower, and 64% of the waterborne contaminants in your blood come through skin absorption. A 10-minute shower can be equivalent to drinking eight glasses of toxic water.[43] All the steam that rolls up contains chlorine and fluoride, which are very toxic chemicals linked to cancer and neurological conditions. Using whole-house filtration, or at least a filter on your shower, is a great way to cut down on the toxic load for you and your family. Look for it online, as this is a very reasonable purchase.

4. Plastics

We live in a plastic world. The environmental hazard we are creating with these harsh chemicals that don't break down is going to catch up with us one day as individuals, and as a planet. Plastics contain disrupting chemicals like xenoestrogens. BPA is an example. Xenoestrogens are hormone-mimicking compounds that can raise estrogen levels in men and women, creating hormone-related diseases and cancers.[44]

Every plastic container has a number found inside a small triangle molded on to it. If you are going to use plastic, it may be beneficial to check the number and avoid certain types.

7 Types of Plastic

1. Polyethylene Terephthalate (PET) Typically this is used in most clear plastic bottles and containers. The issue with it, however, is that it tends to hold food stains, which means food can get caught up in its pores and attract bacteria. #1 plastic also contains antimony trioxide, which is a potential carcinogen. Heating this plastic may leach it into your food—yet another reason I avoid microwaves! So if you are using #1, don't reuse it—recycle it, and certainly don't heat it.
2. High-density Polyethylene (HDPE) is opaque and used in most milk and juice jugs, detergent, butter containers, and toiletries containers. It is generally considered safe, has a low risk of leaching, and can be recycled.
3. Polyvinyl Chloride (PVC) is durable and used in plumbing, food wrap, cooking oil bottles, shower curtains, and inflatable mattresses. Although tough in terms of strength, it is not considered safe for cooking or heating. It commonly contains xenoestrogens and hormone disruptors like

phthalates. I would never heat it and try to avoid skin contact with any products made from it.

4. Low-density Polyethylene (LDPE) is your classic grocery bag and bread bags. The big concern is they are not typically recyclable, so these are very hard on the environment. Go for paper bags.

5. This is polypropylene (PP). It is considered a safe plastic, although I would still avoid heating it. It is found in most condiment bottles, yogurt cups, medicine bottles, and kitchenware. It is recyclable.

6. Polystyrene or Styrofoam commonly found in packing material and disposable food containers. When heated, research shows it leaches toxic chemicals. Reheating food in a to-go container makes for a toxic mistake. Ideally, avoid Styrofoam at all costs.

7. Other Resins mean "everything else", and are often made of a combination of plastics. This means we don't really know what is in them. This category is where BPA is found the most. Plastic store receipts and some coffee cups are made from this. The receipts are especially high in BPA. I opt for no receipts as much as I can, to avoid this hormone disruptor.

To sum it up, plastics #2, #4, #5 keep the body alive. #1, #3, #6, #7 are an early trip to heaven. Ok, that might be a tad extreme, but I would not heat the latter, and would strongly caution against their use. Opt for a water filter and a glass bottle to cut out plastic for you and the environment. Be conscious of what kind of plastic is going into your mouth, what plastic is coming into contact with your skin, and what plastic is in contact with your food. Use glass containers for cooking, food storage, and, ideally, avoid the microwave. Don't get paper/plastic receipts—opt for the email instead, and use paper bags instead of plastic.[44]

The more you can go with glass and other types of non-plastic, the better off you are. Leave a good footprint on the earth and help out your filters too.

5. Fix Your Filters

Avoiding toxins is one thing, but getting the built-up toxins out of you is another. Detoxing should be done regularly. I recommend doing some sort of detox every quarter for your body, especially if you are losing weight because the fat in your body contains a lot of toxins. When you burn fat, you release all those toxins into your system. You want to make sure you're pulling them out of you while you're losing weight so they don't resettle somewhere else and re-toxify you.

There are two types of detoxification, intracellular and extracellular. Your body is equipped with some amazing detoxifying systems—the kidneys, liver, skin, digestive system, lungs, lymph system, and fat cells. They are all built to eliminate toxins.

Intracellular detox refers to the removal of the toxins that reside deep in the organs. These toxins are harder to remove, which means you have to have mechanisms and detox systems that break through the barriers of cells and organs to get deep into the tissues of your brain, lungs, and digestive system in order to suck those toxins from the body. A primary body detoxifier that does this is glutathione; it's our body's street sweeper to get deep into the system and pull these toxins out.

Extracellular detox refers to removing the toxins outside of the cells and organs, such as those in the bloodstream and the digestive system. Many detox solutions just focus extracellularly to pull toxins out through the skin or flush the blood or digestive system. Juice cleanses, fasting, Epsom salt baths, and saunas all extracellularly remove the toxins from the body.

*True detoxification needs
a good one-two punch.*

First, you need to do a deep intracellular detox of the cells and organs, pulling all toxins into the blood and digestive systems. Second, you need to do an extracellular detox to flush them completely out of the body so they don't just re-toxify somewhere else. Without a process that accomplishes both, you will miss many of the toxins in the body, and they can lead to long-term problems.

On a daily regimen, I take greens that contain spirulina, chlorella, and superfoods which are great intracellular detoxifiers that help to build up my body's street sweeper glutathione. Also, I take ample omegas and real salt to keep inflammation and congestion down in my system so the cells can be detoxed. Monthly or quarterly I do extended fasts or have days in which I just drink juices and teas to flush out my system and give it a cleanse. Check out the workbook section at the back of this book to get started. If you have significant toxin concerns, contact a knowledgeable natural doctor to get personal guidance.

Is your body a toxic dump? Step one is to minimize your toxic load, and step two is to properly rid yourself of the toxins already in your body. There are many toxins to avoid or eliminate in order to experience real health, and it may seem daunting to try to cut them out completely. However, the five steps above are a good start. Pair them with your other fixes, and you will greatly minimize your toxicity.

After these last several chapters, I hope it's obvious that when you are clear on what a human body requires to function, it works the way it's supposed to—healthy! Health should be normal, not disease! Fix your focus, fix your food, fix your fitness, fix your frame, and fix your filters. It's like giving a plant water, soil, sunlight, and carbon dioxide. It thrives. And you will too! The only thing in your way now is you. Commit to getting the health that you deserve.

Let's bring this Livingood Daily Formula together and get started.

GRANDMA CUT HER BLOOD PRESSURE MEDICATIONS IN HALF, AND GRANDSON NOW SLEEPS THROUGH THE NIGHT, NO MORE ADENOID FLARE UPS, HASN'T BEEN SICK SINCE BEING UNDER CARE!

NO MORE LUPUS, NORMAL BLOOD PRESSURE, STOMACH IS BETTER, NO MORE HEADACHES AND DIDN'T GO TO THE HOSPITAL FOR OVER A YEAR.

At THC we are giving Olympic and Professionals the same care you are receiving!

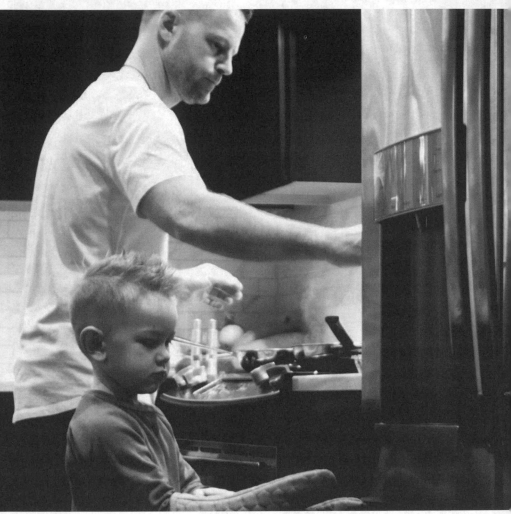

"I'm not telling you it's going to be easy, I'm telling you it's going to be worth it."
– Art Williams

"The two greatest days in your life are the day you are born and the day you find out why.
- Mark Twain

CHAPTER TEN

1% PROGRESS TO LIVINGOOD DAILY

By the time my dad was 53, he'd been given 15 different drugs. My family had experienced over $200,000 in medical expenses and bills. My dad was hardly able to get out of bed, he wasn't working at all, our family was experiencing incredible hardship, and my mom and dad couldn't enjoy the life they were created to live.

After two years of traveling between almost 15 different doctors and specialists, we were expecting my dad to achieve health and go back to normalcy. When you are expecting to get health, but you go to doctors whose only job is to identify, treat, and monitor sickness and disease, you cannot get health. We were doing the same thing over and over—expecting health care, but getting sick care. When you do the same thing over and over and you expect a different result, that's the definition of insanity.

If you want health, you've got to build health; if you want sickness and disease, then manage and treat your sickness and disease, but don't expect health if all you're going to do is wait to get sick and treat your sickness with drugs and surgeries—it's not what the system is designed to do.

Our medical system is designed for emergency care. If you have a car accident, thank God we have helicopters, ambulances, and surgeons. If you have a heart attack, thank God we have medications and surgeries to save lives in a crisis. But, when it comes to building health, you cannot use the current medical system to do it. Until you realize that, your health, the health of your family, and the health of our country will never change. We decided to focus on building health for dad. I flew my dad across the country and moved him into our little apartment with me and my now wife. First, we fixed our focus. It was time to focus on building health, changing his state, less stress, and being grateful for what was good.

We fixed his food, taught him how to shop, and gave him the same recipes you have in this book. We did 10-minute workouts daily at a local football field and fixed his fitness. We started fixing his filters and detoxing his body. Finally, we started to care for his frame. For years he had beat up not only his knees, shoulders, wrists, and hands, but also his spine.

Daily we would rehab his spine and stop the damage by focusing on proper posture while he sat and slept. His range of motion was partially restored, his inflammation decreased, his nervous system began to open up, and within weeks we began seeing massive change.

We focused on improving 1% every day—1% better nutrition choices, 1% better mental health, 1% more gratitude, 1% more movement, 1% less toxicity, 1% better state. 1%. 1%. 1%. If you do that for 21 days, you are 21% better with that area of your health. Imagine if you kept working on small changes for 90 days or 10 years?

I'll never forget the day my father walked into my room and handed me a box. Inside were 15 different pill bottles. I asked, "What is this?"

He said, "I don't need them anymore," and my dad never looked back. He was sent home off all meds shortly afterward. He went biking with my mom again, I went fishing with him again, he saw my wife and I get married, and he saw his first two grandbabies born, my nephews Tristan and Cannon. His life was restored. He got the chance to live good again.

Now It's Your Turn

It doesn't matter if you're young or old, healthy or sick. It doesn't matter how bad your prognosis is or if you've lost all hope. If you are still breathing, then the greatest doctor in the world is still in you.

Maybe you think your health is pretty good. You are the one I worry about the most. My dad's health was "good" the day before his heart shut down. You don't want your biggest asset just to be "good." You want your health to be excellent!

So what is your body trying to tell you? Below is a list of warning signs that indicate that you may have damage already. Circle ANY you may have had in the last 6 months.

Fibromyalgia	Thyroid Problems
Neck Pain	Asthma
Back Pain	High Blood Pressure
Numbness / Tingling	High Cholesterol
Allergies / Sinuses	Headaches
Sleep Problems	Fatigue
Weight Problems	Depression
Digestion / Reflux	Concentration
Multiple Sclerosis	Dizziness
Diabetes	Reproductive Problems
Frequent Colds	Autoimmune Disease

Did you circle some? Have you experienced multiple issues? These are just the common ones plaguing our country. Keep in mind that my dad would not have marked any of these warning signs. He had no idea that he was days or months away from losing his life by losing his health.

If you have one of these symptoms, you have a GIFT! You might call me crazy, but your body is TELLING YOU something is wrong. My dad never got that luxury. You do! Are you listening? Or are you just masking the symptom and ignoring your body's cry for help!?

I truly believe that the reason we've won Top Primary Care Physician and dozens of other awards in our area for several years and have helped over 100,000 people all over the country overcome their conditions—becoming medication-free and canceling surgeries—is that we don't practice sick care, we start by building health.

Why are more doctors not leading you to build health? Have you ever had a physical and had the doctor say you should exercise and eat better? THANKS, DOC. BRILLIANT. Why are we as doctors not HELPING people do exactly that. If we say it's important, then our time should go towards it. You do what you value.

So why is it that our doctors and hospitals are not leading and mandating that people take better care of themselves? If we can mandate a mask or vaccine, why not mandate nutrition and exercise? One simple reason: follow the money. What you have to understand about today's healthcare system is that when you get sick or have an ailment, you become a customer. In order to enter the system, you have to have a disease. Once you get a disease, you're given a drug or offered a surgery—there is no incentive to get you healthy.

Nothing can be done in our current sick care system if you don't have a condition. This has brought forth disease mongering. The number of possible conditions and diagnoses has exploded in recent years because the more conditions and diagnoses there are to treat, the more drugs and surgeries can be given, thus more profit ending up in the pharmaceutical company's pockets. Detach from what your disease is called and start fixing the cause of it.

Now, this isn't your doctor's fault. They're just caught in the middle trying to help people and make a difference, but the only two tools they're given to work with are medications and surgeries. Neither are they given any incentive to get people off drugs; in fact, they are given incentives to keep them on! I still believe that if our job and passion are to see people become healthy, we should be stepping up.

The measure of a doctor should not be by how many people he/she put on drugs but by how many he/she helped get off drugs and stay off.

You cannot remove an organ and make someone healthier. You cannot add a toxin to a body and make it healthier. You may save a life from a crisis, but it does not build health.

No drug or chemical that man could come up with could ever come close to mimicking the power of the doctor on the inside. So, what I'm saying is that there's no incentive for any pharmaceutical company or any hospital that makes their entire livelihood off of sick people taking drugs and surgeries to ever come up with anything to take care of or eliminate your ailments. There's no incentive for them to do it. It doesn't mean they don't care about people; it just means there's no incentive for them to drive such a cause.

Medicine will never do research studies to come up with a way to eliminate your disease. There will be no research dollars, walks around tracks, or 5K's for daily stress reduction habits and real-food eating. There's no big money in equipping you to be your own doctor.

As a doctor, the first place I always start is simply building health. In fact, I got to a point that I wouldn't even do a consultation until a person has read this book and applied it for at least 21 days. Why? Not because I don't care about them, but because I care too much.

Plus, I don't think the consultation is even necessary. 80% of problems disappear when the foundations of health are applied, and therefore I would have been treating or addressing something that just needed some simple health. Livingood Daily is a movement to lead the masses of people through actually building health. Not one at a time, but together. Not just talking about it or making a suggestion, but actually getting in the trenches and doing it. Focus on sickness and disease, and you get sickness and disease. Focus on building health, and you get health.

The urgency of NOW.

My dad followed the steps in this book, and it saved his life. We experienced five more amazing years with my father. He got to see me get married, meet and watch his first two grandbabies growing up, and go biking with my mom again. I went fishing with my dad again, and we had life conversations, moments, and memories that no one can ever take away from me.

However, he got this message too late. It is why I write with such passion and urgency. Dad needed this book 30 years ago. In 2013, at age 58, my dad passed away. The interference of prolonged nerve damage and years on heavy drugs shut my father's liver down. He left behind my mom, to whom he'd been married for over 30 years—they were high school sweethearts. He left behind my brother and his wife, me and my wife, and six grandbabies; four of the grandbabies he never met—including all 3 of my kids—Sullivan, London, and Ireland.

I believe there was more potential there for my dad, but his time was cut short. God uses all things for good. I would love to still have my father around, but I believe God gave me the second-best thing out of all of this, and that is a purpose.

*The biggest test of my family's life—
my dad's struggles, disease, and the hardship
we went through—turned into the biggest
testimony of our lives.*

Thousands of people just like you are now being helped all across the world. My wife, mom, brother, sister-in-law, and I all now work virtually and in clinics, striving every day to save people from ever going down the road our family traveled, teaching these principles.

The two greatest days in your life are the day you are born and the day you find out why.

My dad's sickness served a purpose. I've personally walked hundreds of thousands of people through the laws of health we've learned and have seen thousands come off of medications, get out of wheelchairs, walk away from walkers, overcome diseases that doctors said they would never overcome, beat cancer and heart disease, overcome the need for oxygen tanks, heal from diabetes, and so much more. We've seen people overcome insurmountable odds and experience real health, we've seen families get healthy together, and we've seen people lose thousands and thousands of pounds. The biggest thing, though, is seeing kids, adults, and families getting healthy before the disease ever shows up so we never even have to experience the tragedies or even the miracle-recovery stories.

This book is for all the potential that comes from people achieving amazing health, which I'll never fully see or be able

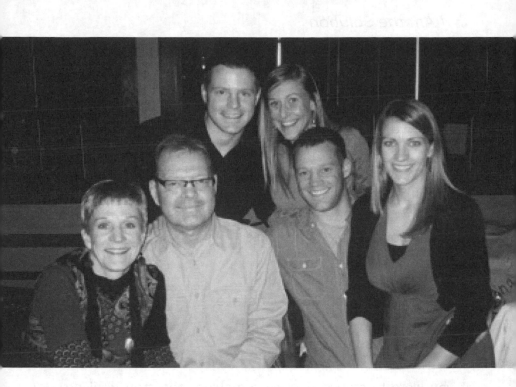

to measure. This book is for the lives that are touched, the miracles that happen, the life changes that can live on, the stories that are written, the songs that are created, the ideas that come to life, the inventions that are realized, and the potential that will come out of people because they have the chance to live good. Their life wasn't cut short unnecessarily, and they didn't suffer needlessly.

All the struggles in your life can be used for good, if you let them. I made a promise to my dad and myself that, as long as I live, I will do everything I can to prevent anyone from going down the road my family had to go down. In order to achieve those results, there are two rally cries that I teach every person who becomes a part of the Livingood Daily movement, ensuring success.

1. *I Am the Solution*

What I learned in biochemistry is that once you have a formula, all you have to do is follow the steps and add a catalyst to create the solution. We would add acid or enzymes, and the solution would occur at a faster rate. A catalyst is a person that precipitates an event. YOU are that catalyst. You have the formula. You have the plan. It's time to be the catalyst for the event of changing your life. You hold the formula's secret to the solution—the Livingood Daily Formula. Here are the first four steps of the five-step formula:

1. Decide that I must change.
2. Appoint myself head of state.
3. Establish the 5 Foundations.
4. Take massive action.

If you were to stop eating, stop moving, and stop drinking, how long would you survive? Not long! Why? Because you have to do your part! You GET to be the catalyst. Put in place the simple foundations of what a human needs to thrive, and give yourself the best chance to experience real health.

The solution you have searched for here so long is sitting in your seat! YOU ARE THE SOLUTION. Believe it. The greatest doctor in the world is in you, and you have the ability to let him or her loose. Here is your mantra. "I am the solution. I am the solution. I am the solution." You have all you need.

I AM THE SOLUTION

You can fix your food. You can fix your fitness. You can fix your focus. You can fix your frame. You can fix your filters. You can be the catalyst.

If you can "lifestyle" your way into it, you can "lifestyle" your way out of it.

If you stand in the street in front of a bus, have good intentions, pray, talk about moving and changing but you don't get your butt out of the way, it won't end well. You have to move! You have to act.

Be careful because sick, drugged, misinformed, ignorant, and lazy is exactly what many people in the world are and what the enemy wants you to be. The world and the negative voices of Sally and Barry in your head want to take away your commitment and discourage you, blindfold you from the truth, uninspire you, distract you, and make you focus on how hard it is. Disease, drugs, and early deaths are hard—health isn't. I didn't say it was going to be easy; I just said it would be worth it.

The Livingood Daily Formula

1. *Decide I must change.*
2. *Appoint myself head of state.*
3. *Establish the 5 Foundations.*
4. *Take massive action.*
5. *Live good daily. Positively reinforce the new habits to make it a lifestyle.*

Get a Strong Room

Growing up in Iowa, the largest wrestling state in the country I naturally became a wrestler. It was incredibly competitive, but I excelled and made several state title runs. To be successful in wrestling in Iowa, you could not do it on your own. The level at which you were able to compete was determined by the strength of your teammates. If you had a room full of lazy teammates that you could slough off with each day, then chances are you never developed the skills to be a champion. If your room was filled with other state qualifiers and committed winners, then you would get better a lot faster and win as well. The most successful wrestlers in the state came from strong rooms.

You need a strong room for your life. A group of people doing, thinking, and committing to winning with their health and life, encouraging each other along the way and picking each other up, even asking each other questions to get better. A strong room makes for much faster and more predictable results.

This is why we made the Livingood Daily Challenge, private groups of people executing the principles of this book together for over 4 weeks. This is what accomplishes the 5th part of the Livingood Daily Formula. Reward and celebrate progress. Let me explain by reviewing the 5-step formula and by explaining how we bring this to life in the challenge groups:

1. We MUST change.

Get a daily reminder and constant reinforcement from me, my team, and a huge community that we MUST commit to change.

2. Head of state.

Each day we teach, motivate, sing, dance, encourage, cry,

celebrate, problem-solve, and protect the one thing that enables us to make the right choices for long term change... our state.

3. 5 Foundations.

Go deeper and actually apply the 5 Foundation Fixes. Fix your focus, food, fitness, frame, and filters in a systematic, easy-to-follow way. Avoid being overwhelmed, and finally, do it.

4. Take massive action.

Research shows that your chances of hitting your goal go up to 95% when you have an accountability partner. In the group, you will have me and several thousand others all going the same way on the journey to help each other out.

5. Reward the new habit and live good daily.

In week 4, we celebrate hundreds of testimonials of people off medications, weight losses of 5-30 pounds, and overcoming conditions of all types. We also vote and crown a challenge champion and award winners.

When you celebrate your new habit, you rewire your brain to WANT to choose it again. This is the moment these new habits become a lifestyle!

The last thing you would want at that point would be to slip back, so we help you turn the Livingood Daily Challenge into the Livingood Daily Lifestyle. This is where we repeat the formula over and over to live good daily.

Visit *www.livingooddaily.com* to learn more about the next

challenge. You do not have to do this alone—how powerful would it be to do it with me and thousands of others?

You are the solution! The formula is set, and now it is just time to execute. Decide that today is the day. Plus, when you commit to be healthy and live good, you give permission for others around you to do the same.

So now that YOU are heading down the right path, begin to think outside of yourself. Who else around you need real health? How can you strengthen your current room? Bring them with you. Do it together.

2. We Are The Solution

There are so many other people around you that haven't heard this message. 99% of people have never had a doctor teach and lead them through actually building health. So many other people are trying programs, products, tests, specialists, supplements, gimmicks, books, self-help tricks, drugs, and "sick care" doctors to try to get their health on track.

—— *Health isn't a program, it's a necessity!* ——

While you're sitting there right now, nod if you thought of one, three, five, or twenty other people that need to hear something that you learned in this book. I ask you to share it with them. What if you gave someone a chance to break free from their chains of disease and live good? Who deserves to know true health principles and the foundations of Livingood daily? Who deserves to have real health care? Who deserves to have a plan to get themselves and their family fully alive? Everybody does.

Family and Friends That Get Healthy Together, Stay Together

Learn this from my dad! Why would you leave your kids and your spouse to suffer the same consequences and the same damage that you did? There have been generational curses that have been passed down long enough—that ends with you right now.

What if you just started with your family? I made the decision that, even though my grandfather had cancer, my grandmother had Alzheimer's, my dad had massive heart problems, and my other grandfather died of heart problems—that these disease patterns end now! I can now lead myself, my family, and my kids down the road of experiencing real health and life to the fullest so we don't have to be a victim of the disease. We can experience real health and achieve our purpose on this earth.

My dad instilled incredible values in my life. He started me on the right path young, and now that I'm older, I don't stray from it. He never understood the value of health, though. I now understand it and keep it as one of the highest values for my kids.

Start your children off on the way they should go, and even when they are old, they will not turn from it.
- Proverbs 22:6

As a constant reminder of what my dad instilled in me and a reminder to do that same thing for my son, my wife gave me a new ring with Proverbs 22:6 inscribed on the inside when my son was born. I share this with you as an assignment: don't leave your children and family behind to suffer the same problems you have.

We hold health in high regard and value in our household. We know we are of less good to our family or our purpose if we are sick or dead. We focus on the light, not the darkness. We focus on building health, not on sickness and disease.

Lead your family. Lead your loved ones. Stop those generational curses—it's not your genes. The Producer didn't screw up; He created you to be healthy, and you can break those generational curses and decide from here on out that your family tree and the family trees around you are going to be healthy—not wither away, crumble, or suffer more. Decide that you're going to uproot your family tree and plant it in healthy soil and that you're going to lead others to do the same.

This book is not for you alone. You are part of something. You are now part of the solution. Together we can be the solution—the solution to a sick, suffering, hurting, and stressed-out world. We can leave it better than we found it. I believe everyone needs this message, and I encourage you to share this book, passing it along to others around you. Get one for your family members as a Christmas or birthday gift.

There's no better gift than the gift of life.

There are so many people on this planet who are suffering

right now. When you have health, you have the world. You could lose everything, but if you are breathing, you have a lot. You can give someone the world by helping them live good.

Imagine how much better our world would be if millions of people were focused on gratitude rather than stress, if people were feeding their bodies real food instead of garbage, if people were moving and energizing their bodies each day with 10-minute workouts. If we had full mobility instead of being sedentary, if we stopped toxifying our bodies, minds, and the world with chemicals, how much happier of a place would it be? How much more work would we accomplish? How much money would we save? How many more life experiences would we have?

Believe in the doctor inside of you, not in what man has painted health care to be. Go "live good" yourself so you can do good in the world. Share this gift with others—other family members, other friends, other church members, and other people in your town, city, and state.

You are the solution for your health, and together **we are the solution** to real health care.

Live good. Do good.

CITATIONS

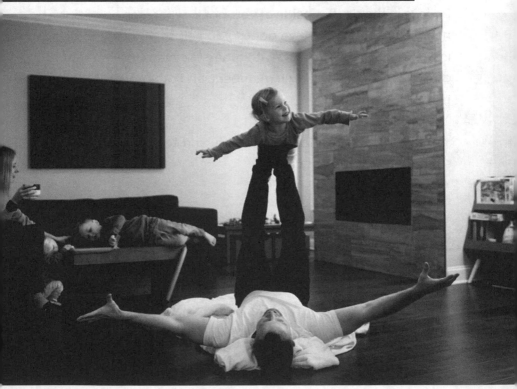

1. "Partnership to Fight Chronic Disease," Almanac of Chronic Disease, (2009).
2. Blue, L. (2012, November 7). Study Shows More Than Half of All Americans Will Get Heart Disease. Retrieved from http://healthland.time.com/2012/11/07/study-shows-more-than-half-of-all-americans-will-get-heart-disease/.
3. National Cancer Institute Stat Fact Sheets. (n.d.). Retrieved November 18, 2015, from http://seer.cancer.gov/statfacts/html/all.html.
4. The world health report 2000 — health systems: improving performance. Geneva: World Health Organization, 2000.
5. America's Health Disadvantage. (n.d.). Retrieved November 18, 2015, from http://www.bestmasterofscienceinnursing.com/health/.
6. Fox, M. (n.d.). More US babies die on their first day than in 68 other countries, report shows – NBC News. Retrieved from http://www.nbcnews.com/health/more-us-babies-die-their-first-day-68-other-countries-6C9700437.
7. Haelle, T. (2014, September 24). U.S. Infant Mortality Rate Worse than other Countries. Retrieved from http://www.cbsnews.com/news/u-s-infant-mortality-rate-worse-than-other-countries/.
8. Geoga.se: Gazetteer – The World – Population – Top 100 By Country (2015). (n.d.). Retrieved November 18, 2015, from http://www.geoba.se/population.php?pc=world&type=15.
9. 5 Ways Our Healthcare System Is Broken. (n.d.). Retrieved November 18, 2015, from http://www.mba-healthcare-management.com/system/.
10. Study Shows 70 Percent of Americans take Prescription drugs. (2013, June 20). Retrieved from http://www.cbsnews.com/news/study-shows-70-percent-of-americans-take-prescription-drugs/.
11. Mathews, A. (2010, December 28). So Young and So Many Pills. Retrieved from http://www.wsj.com/articles/SB10001424052970203731004576046073896 4/5588
12. Smith, R. (Ed.). (1991, October 5). Where is the Wisdom? The Poverty of Medical Evidence. Retrieved November 18, 2015, from http://www.chiro.org/LINKS/FULL/Where_Is_The_Wisdom.shtml.
13. Null, G., et al. (2010). Death by Medicine. Mount Jackson, VA: Praktikos Books.
14. Tamkins, T. (2009, June 5). Medical Bills Prompt more than 60 Percent of U.S. Bankruptcies. Retrieved from http://www.cnn.com/2009/HEALTH/06/05/bankruptcy.medical.bills/.
15. Cowitt, B. (2010, June 7). Starbucks CEO: "We spend more on health care than coffee" Retrieved from http://archive.fortune.com/2010/06/07/news/companies/starbucks_schultz_healthcare.fortune/index.htm.
16. Volksy, I. (2008, November 18). The AutoMakers and the HealthCare Crisis. Retrieved from http://thinkprogress.org/health/2008/11/18/170556/auto-health/.
17. Kilo CM, Larson EB. Exploring the harmful effects of health care. JAMA, 2009;302(1):89-91.
18. North Carolina State Public Health Statistics. America's Health Rankings. (n.d.). Retrieved November 18, 2015, from http://www.americashealthrankings.org/NC.
19. Proeschold-Bell, R. J., LeGrand, S., James, J., Wallace, A., Adams, C., & Toole, D. (2009). A theoretical model of the holistic health of United Methodist clergy. Journal of Religion and Health, DOI 10.1007/s10943-009- 9250-1.
20. About WHO. (n.d.). Retrieved November 18, 2015, from http://www.who.int/about/en/.
21. Sharpless SK: "Susceptibility of spinal roots to compression block." The

Research Status of Spinal Manipulative Therapy. NINCDS monograph 15, DHEW publication (NIH) 76-998:155, 1975.

22. Kent, C. (1995, December 1). Nerve Compression Physiology. Retrieved from http://www.subluxation.com/nerve-compression-physiology/.

23. Kelly, M. (1956). Is Pain Due to Pressure on Nerves?: Spinal Tumors and the Intervertebral Disk. Neurology, 32-36.

24. Ehrlich, S. (n.d.). Atherosclerosis. Retrieved from http://umm.edu/health/medical/altmed/condition/atherosclerosis.

25. http://www.kidney.org.au/.

26. Average Drug Label Lists Over Whopping 70 Side Effects. (2011, June 9). Retrieved from http://articles.mercola.com/sites/articles/archive/2011/06/09/average-drug-label-lists-over-whopping-70-side-effects.aspx.

27. Popping Pills: Prescription Drug Abuse in America. (2014, January 2). Retrieved November 18, 2015, from http://www.drugabuse.gov/related-topics/trends-statistics/infographics/popping-pills-prescription-drug-abuse-in-america.

28. 100 Very Cool Facts About the Human Body [Web log post]. (2008, February 27). Retrieved November 18, 2015, from http://icantseeyou.typepad.com/my_weblog/2008/02/100-very-cool-f.html and http://graphs.net/top-10-human-body-infographics.html.

29. 18 Amazing Facts About the Human Body – Infographic. (n.d.). Retrieved November 18, 2015, from http://www.advancedphysicalmedicine.org/18-amazing-facts-human-body-infographic.php.

30. Russell, Matthew E B, et al. "Inclusion of a Rest Period in Diaphragmatic Breathing Increases High-Frequency Heart Rate Variability: Implications for Behavioral Therapy." Psychophysiology, U.S. National Library of Medicine, Mar. 2017, www.ncbi.nlm.nih.gov/pmc/articles/PMC5319881/#R27.

31. Glassman SD, Bridwell K, Dimar JR, Horton W, Berven S, Schwab F (2005) The impact of positive sagittal balance in adult spinal deformity. Spine 30(18):2024–2029.

32. Research shows that a loss or increase in spinal curves increases mortality (speeds up death) and takes up to 14 years off your life. J. BONE JOINT SURG. AM 1981 June; 63(5):702-12. Weinstein Sh, Zavala DC, Ponseti IV.

33. Kapandji. (n.d.). "For every inch of Forward Head Posture, it can increase the weight of the head on the spine by an additional 10 pounds." -Kapandji, Physiology of Joints, Vol. 3.

34. Candeo, N. (2014, November 19). Study: Texting can put 60 pounds of pressure on the spine, lead to possible surgery. Retrieved from http://www.syracuse.com/news/index.ssf/2014/11/texting_spine_study_pressure_60_pounds.html.

35. "The mortality rate (with AIS)(Adolescent Idiopathic Scoliosis) is 15 %". "Individuals with Scoliosis life expectancy is decreased by 14 years": idiopathic scoliosis: long term follow-up and prognosis in untreated patients. J.Bone Joint Surg Am 1981 Jun;63(5):702-12.

36. Chandrasekhar, K, et al. "A Prospective, Randomized Double-Blind, Placebo-Controlled Study of Safety and Efficacy of a High-Concentration Full-Spectrum Extract of Ashwagandha Root in Reducing Stress and Anxiety in Adults." Indian Journal of Psychological Medicine, Medknow Publications & Media Pvt Ltd, July 2012, www.ncbi.nlm.nih.gov/pmc/articles/PMC3573577/.

37. Shimizu, K. MD., Nakamura, M. MD., Nishikawa, Y. MD., Hijikata, S. MD., Chiba, K. MD., Toyama, Y MD. (2005). Urgent Need for Normal Curves. Spine, Volume 30 (21). Pp 2388-2392.

38. U.S. Sugar Consumption: A Not-So-Sweet Reality – Dental CE Courses: The Richmond Institute. (n.d.). Retrieved November 18, 2015, from http://

www.richmondinstitute.com/u-s-consumption-of-sugar-a-not-so-sweet-reality.
39. Chang, C., Ke, D., Chen, J. (2009). Essential Fatty Acids and Human Brain. Acta Neurol Taiwan. Volume 18 (4): 23 1-41.
40. Mercola, J. (2012, February 10). Peak Fitness Exercises Benefits. Retrieved November 18, 2015, from http://fitness.mercola.com/sites/fitness/archive/2012/02/10/phil-campbell-interview.aspx.
41. Mercola, J. (2012, June 1). Long Cardio Workout Dangers. Retrieved from http://fitness.mercola.com/sites/fitness/archive/2012/06/01/long-cardio-workout-dangers.aspx,
42. Mercola, J. (2011, May 5). How to Make Sure You Burn Calories for Hours after Your Workout. Retrieved from http://fitness.mercola.com/sites/fitness/archive/2011/05/05/how-to-make-sure-you-burn-calories-for-hours-after-your-workout.aspx.
43. Michaelis, K. (n.d.). Chlorinated Showers & Baths Kill Gut Flora. Retrieved November 18, 2015, from http://www.foodrenegade.com/chlorinated-showers-baths-kill-gut-flora/
44. Dirty Dozen Endocrine Disruptors. (2013, October 28). Retrieved from http://www.ewg.org/research/dirty-dozen-list-endocrine-disruptors.
45. Longo, Valter D, and Mark P Mattson. "Fasting: Molecular Mechanisms and Clinical Applications." Cell Metabolism, U.S. National Library of Medicine, 4 Feb. 2014, www.ncbi.nlm.nih.gov/pmc/articles/PMC3946160/.
46. HD;, Davis DR; Epp MD; Riordan. "Changes in USDA Food Composition Data for 43 Garden Crops, 1950 to 1999." Journal of the American College of Nutrition, U.S. National Library of Medicine, 2004, pubmed.ncbi.nlm.nih.gov/15637215/.

All bible verses are from the New International Version (NIV).

CITATIONS

ACKNOWLEDGEMENTS

I couldn't end without saying "thank you" to so many people who have made the journey possible to this point. First, and most importantly, I thank God for His grace and using all things for good to help me find my purpose. Second, my wife--I tear up just writing about you; you're the love of my life, my best friend, and God's biggest blessing to me. Thanks for giving me permission to be me--I love you. Third, my family for raising me right, pushing through the hard times, and enjoying the good times. Fourth, the dear friends who helped me put this all together and their unwavering support. Finally, to the best clinic, team, and patients in the world... you make every day a joy. Health care needs to change—we have a lot of work to do!

GO
MAKE IT A GREAT DAY;
YOU MIGHT AS WELL
YOU'LL NEVER GET IT BACK.
LIVE GOOD!

SUPPLEMENTS
101

YOUR COMPREHENSIVE GUIDE TO SUPPLEMENTS

Get all of the information you need to fully understand which supplements you should take for your condition and which supplements you should avoid.

1. Rancid Oils

Hydrogenated oils congest the cells and negatively impact cholesterol, antioxidants, and inflammation. Oils to avoid are soybean, safflower, sunflower, cottonseed, vegetable, canola, and palm oil. The 2010 Dietary Guidelines for Americans specifically states: "Keep trans fatty acid consumption as low as possible by limiting foods that contain synthetic sources of trans fats, such as partially hydrogenated oils, and by limiting other solid fats."

Selecting supplements with stable, strong naturally occurring oils avoids this negative impact. These oils include coconut, avocado, olive, macadamia, borage, flaxseed, grapeseed, and fish oil.

About fish oil and flaxseed oil knowledge of the supplement companies' process to protect these fragile oils is highly recommended. Refrigerated versions (optional), added vitamin E or tocopherols, and dark-colored bottles are three ways this is done. Buying large bulk bottles of fish oil is not advised as they are not protected and easily go rancid.

2. Heavy Metals

Lead, mercury, and aluminum are linked to neurological disorders, inflammation, and heart dysfunction. It is crucial to finding supplements that test for and reduce heavy metal exposure.

For example, your fish oil choice should test or state that they are "Molecularly distilled and 3rd-party tested to ensure PCBs, dioxins, mercury, lead, and other contaminants are below acceptable limits set by the Council for Responsible Nutrition and other advisory agencies."

3. Added Sugar, Artificial Sugars and Hidden Sugars

We typically consume 152 pounds of sugar per person, per year, in America, according to the Department of Health and Human Services. To help avoid such excessive intake, choose supplements with no added sugar.

Beware of maltodextrin, any form of starch, any word ending in -ose (sucrose, glucose, etc), corn products, potato products, rice products, or any other forms of sugar. Also avoid toxic forms of artificial flavorings (Sucralose, aspartame, Splenda, Nutrasweet, etc.).

NOTE: Cellulose (fiber) and allulose (sugar alcohol) are acceptable.

4. Artificial Colorings
- FD&C Blue Nos. 1 & 2
- FD&C Green No. 3
- FD&C Red Nos. 3 & 40
- FD&C Yellow Nos. 5 & 6
- Caramel

The only purpose of artificial colorings is to make the supplement look more appealing or fun. This is solely for marketing purposes, to cover up the poor quality of the supplement, and does not help your health. The FDA itself has shown a connection between artificial food dyes and behavior issues, ADHD, and hyperactivity.

5. Synthetic Vitamins

Healthy-food forms of vitamins are very important for proper health. However, synthetic/fortified vitamins are created using chemical compounds that are not found in nature. Your body cannot utilize them as they can natural vitamins sourced from food. According to the Organic Consumers Association, fat-soluble vitamins (A, D, E & K) are especially dangerous in synthetic form, as they can build up in your body's fat tissues and liver. These along with fortified vitamins should be avoided. Look for methylated B vitaminn, Vitamin D3 instead of D2, Vitamin E in the tocotrienol form as opposed to tocopherol, and avoid synthetic forms of Vitamin C made from corn.

6. Toxic Additives

- Magnesium Silicate: Used as a filler and anti-caking agent. Tied to lung problems when inhaled, often contaminated with asbestos in the mining process, and suspected to cause problems when ingested.
- Magnesium Stearate / Stearic Acid: The stearic acid used to make preservatives is sometimes taken from cottonseed, canola, or palm oil. A vegetable source is advised.
- Sodium Benzoate: Benzene-based chemicals have been linked to various cancers. Sodium benzoate can form benzene if it's taken with toxic ascorbic acid. According to the US National Library of Medicine National Institutes of Health, sodium benzoate has the potential to damage cells and DNA.
- Titanium Dioxide: Titanium dioxide has been shown to cause lung inflammation & compromise the immune system.
- Arsenic and Carrageenan can also be potential sources of toxicity.

Look For Toxin Free Guarantees:

- Gluten-Free

- Dairy-Free
- Soy-Free
- Egg-Free
- No Yeast
- No MSG
- No Preservatives
- No Artificial Colorings
- No Artificial Flavorings
- Sourced From Grass-Fed, Free Range, and Wild-Caught (When Applicable)
- No Heavy Metals
- No GMOs

Dr. Livingood's Cheat Sheet For Supplements By Condition

Supplements are just that—"supplements." They are never meant to treat. Step one before any supplement is to do the Livingood Daily Challenge to build real health every day. You don't HAVE to do any of these to be healthy; it just makes things easier or supports a condition.

Inflammation:
- Omegas (3,6,7 and 9) - 400mg - 2400mg Daily
- Turmeric 500mg - 3g Daily
- Livingood Daily Greens 1 - 2 Scoops Per Day

Immune Support:
- Vitamin D3 2,000-20,000 ius per day depending on the case. Take with K1, K2 (MK4 & MK7), Mg, Vitamins A and E, and Take With Fat To Absorb (Livingood Daily Vitamin D)
- Vitamin C with Quercetin 1,500-10,000mg per day depending on the case (High-Dose Vitamin C or Livingood Daily Energyze)

- Vitamin B6 (Methylated) (Livingood Daily Collagen+Multi or Livingood Daily Multivitamin)
- Zinc 10-50mg per day (Livingood Daily Vitamin D and Collagen +Multi)
- Oregano Oil + Monolaurin (Used for a fungus or virus)
- Silver Serum (Colloidal Silver) (Used for bacteria and infections)
- Probiotics (Livingood Daily Greens and Vitamin D)

Gut Health Support:
- L- Glutamine, Collagen, and Probiotics (Livingood Daily Greens and Collagen+Multi)

Liver Supplements:
- Spirulina, Chlorella, Fruits, and Veggies (Livingood Daily Greens)
- Milk Thistle (Livingood Daily Collagen+Multi)

Thyroid Health Support:
- Selenium, Iodine, Methylated B Vitamins (Livingood Daily Thyroid Support)

Heart:
- High Blood Pressure
  » Hawthorne, Potassium, Magnesium, Lipoic Acid, Pomegranate, Beet Root Powder (Livingood Daily Healthy Blood Pressure Support)
  » Omega 3, 6, 7, and 9 Fish-and-Plant-Based (Livingood Daily Omegas+Turmeric)
- Cholesterol
  » Plant Sterols, Beta Glucan, Grape Seed Extract, Curcumin, Reduced CoQ10, Garlic, Vitamin E (Livingood Daily Cholesterol Support)
  » Omegas 3, 6, 7, and 9 Fish and Plant-Based with

Turmeric (Livingood Daily Omegas+Turmeric)

- Afib/Electircal Issues
  - » Taurine, D-Ribose and Electrolytes (Livingood Daily Energyze)
  - » Methylated B Vitamins (Livingood Daily Collagen+Multi or Livingood Dialy Multivitamin)
  - » Green Foods, Potassium, and Anti-Inflammatories (Livingood Daily Greens)
- Heart Valve Issues
  - » Vitamin D3 taken with K1, K2 (MK4 & MK7), Mg, Vitamins A and E, and Take With Fat To Absorb (Livingood Daily Vitamin D)
  - » Vitamin C as a precursor for collagen for blood vessels (Livingood Daily Energyze)
  - » Livingood Daily Greens
- Atherosclerosis/Angina
  - » High Potency Omegas 1500mg+ (Livingood Daily Omegas+Turmeric)
  - » Plant Sterols, Beta Glucan, Grape Seed Extract, Curcumin, Reduced CoQ10, Garlic, Vitamin E (Livingood Daily Cholesterol Support)
  - » Vitamin K taken as K1, K2 (MK4 & MK7), Mg, Vitamins A, D, and E (Livingood Daily Vitamin D or Multi)

Blood Sugar/Diabetes Support:
- Glucomannan (Livingood Daily Collagen+Multi Protein)
- Juice Fasting and Meal Replacements (Livingood Daily Greens)
- Livingood Daily Bars

Allergies Support:
- Nettles, Tinospora, and Quercetin (Livingood Daily Allergen Support)

Everyday Supplement Recommendations:

The below supplements are what I use every day. Take what you would like but many just like to know—"What is the doctor using?"

- Vitamin D3 taken with K1, K2 (MK4 & MK7), Mg, Vitamins A and E, and take with fat to absorb (Livingood Daily Vitamin D)
- Livingood Daily Collagen+Multi Protein - My multi plus blood sugar support
- Omegas 3, 6, 7, and 9 Fish and Plant-based with Turmeric (Livingood Daily Omegas+Turmeric)
- Livingood Daily Greens with 54+ Nutrients, Probiotics, and Digestive Enzymes
- BONUS: Livingood Daily Energyze for Vitamin C and Electrolyte Powder
- BONUS: Livingood Daily Bars as Snacks or Healthy Meals

Remember, every day the most important thing you can do is eat real food, move for at least 10 minutes, breathe, de-stress, and avoid toxins by doing the challenge. Once those foundations are in place, then use supplements to add to your health.

Live Good!
Dr. Livingood

LIVINGOOD DAILY CHALLENGE WORKBOOK

DR. LIVINGOOD

LETTER FROM DR. LIVINGOOD

What is the biggest asset you have?

America takes 75% of the world's medications and seven out of ten people die of chronic and preventable diseases. The health care system meant to remedy this problem is now the third leading cause of death itself. This exists because we often ignore our health or assume we are healthy until disease hits. Then once disease hits we manage the sickness with drugs and surgeries. That's not health care, that's sick care. We have a giant sick care system.

My father fell victim to this sick care system and lost his health at age 51. When he lost his biggest asset he never worked again, couldn't bike, fish, enjoy his family, and we endured over $200,000 in medical bills. This drove me to find an answer for him. My dad didn't need more drugs and surgeries, he needed health. The principles in this challenge are what saved his life. Then I conducted my own double-blind research study on how that system of real health would work for others. We have now guided over 25,000 people in my clinic and around the world to follow this proven method to feel healthy, get off medications, overcome disease, lose the weight, and experience real health.

SO WHAT IS THE SOLUTION?

Your stomach acid can dissolve razor blades, your lungs have a surface area as large as a tennis court, your brain has enough electricity to light up a 10 watt light bulb, and your heart will give off enough power in the next 24 hours to lift 3 fully loaded greyhound buses off of the ground. With the level of power and intellegence in YOU, the greatest doctor in the world is not at Mayo Clinic or Harvard, the greatest doctor in the world is YOU. Just give your body what it needs and fix your health.

Fix your food through real nutrition. Fix your fitness in 10 minutes per day. Fix your focus by building health and beating stress. Fix your filters by detoxing. If you want health, and focus on the activities of building health, that is how you will experience real health. You are the solution! Stop focusing on the problems and start focusing on the solution. Every day empower yourself to know...

I AM THE SOLUTION!

The steps in this workbook will begin to lead you through a 21-day challenge to build health, beat disease, eliminate medications, lose weight, lose stress, and regain LIFE. The answer you are looking for is right inside of you. You just have to do it.

YOU ARE THE SOLUTION!

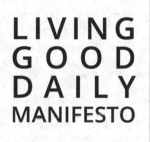

LIVING
GOOD
DAILY
MANIFESTO

I TAKE RESPONSIBILITY FOR MY **HEALTH**. TODAY I CHOOSE GRATITUDE & A **SMILE**. HEALTH TASTES SWEETER THAN MY CRAVINGS. **I EAT TO LIVE** NOT LIVE TO EAT. MY 10 MINUTE WORKOUTS ENERGIZE ME. I WILL NOT WAIT FOR SICKNESS AND DISEASE. **I CHOOSE TO BUILD HEALTH**. I WILL ACCOMPLISH A LIFE CHANGING SHIFT IN MY HEALTH & **HELP OTHERS** DO THE SAME. THE GREATEST DOCTOR IN THE WORLD IS ME. I WILL NEVER GET TODAY BACK. **I CHOOSE TO LIVE GOOD**.

#IAMTHESOLUTION

WHAT'S YOUR DESTINATION

We are all on a journey to experience real health. Unfortunately the only vehicle most use to try and get there is drugs, surgeries, and yearly testing. That vehicle is not designed to get you healthy, it's built as an emergency vehicle. What you now hold is the manual on how to begin to drive your new vehicle. A vehicle that will help you build towards REAL health. We will be your guides but you have to drive. Before you drive you must know where you are going. The first question is WHERE is your destination? What does real health mean for you? What are your health goals and what do you need to do to get there? Let's "pop the hood" before we take off and understand the engine that will be powering your journey...

WHAT IS MY WORD? _____

WHAT AM I STOPPING? _____

WHAT AM I STARTING? _____

WHO AM I DOING IT FOR? _____

WHAT ARE MY REAL HEALTH GOALS?

_____

_____

_____

_____

_____

_____

_____

_____

_____

Commitment Statement

I, _____ , am committed to
the Livingood Daily Lifestyle and am ready
to start experiencing REAL health! I am not
going to wait for sickness and disease or
settle for a diagnosis. Instead, I will focus on
building REAL health and making it simple!

#IAMTHESOLUTION

5 Fixes of Real Health

There are 5 areas to fix and work on when it comes to health...

FOOD

The goal will be to eat only real food and give your system a complete break. You'll learn how to do this by cutting sugar, cranking up the fat, cleaning up the protein, and caring about nutrients.

FITNESS

The simplest, most efficient way to kill disease, lose weight, and experience real health is by moving your body. When it comes to optimal function of your body, it's all about high intensity and shorter duration. Teach your body how be a fat-burner and get in shape fast with the 10-Minute Workout.

FOCUS

If you focus on finding and managing sickness and disease, you get sickness and disease. If you focus on building health, you get health. Fix your focus and change your life. Each day get inspired, reduce stress, and get perspective to focus on experience real health.

FILTERS

It's impossible to avoid all toxins but two major things can be done to detox your body. Each day reduce toxin exposure in your life and optimize your bodies filters (liver, kidneys, gut, etc.) to remove the toxins already in you.

FRAME

Your body is your home. If you wear it out where will you live? Your joints make up your frame and protect your organs, nervous system, and most important body parts. Learning to rehab and take care of these joints ensures they do not fail you or restrict you from daily living.

CHALLENGE FOOD GUIDELINES

Cut THE SUGAR

Research shows that the average American eats around 130 pounds of sugar every year! When you compare that to the turn of the 19th Century in America, an individual ate less than 20 pounds a year. Sugar is in everything! Why? It tastes sweeter, so you eat more. Food companies know this, and they are exploiting this all the way to the grave. Sugar is an anti-nutrient—not only does it harm you, but it also takes up space for needed nutrients. It all has to go for now!

The first initial response I get to that statement is, "I don't eat that much sugar, Dr. Livingood." Yes, you do. Understand that I'm writing this right now to a world of sugar addicts. When you try to tell someone that they are an addict, often times, they don't want to hear it.

It's said that sugar is more addictive to the brain than cocaine is, so I do realize the challenge when I start messing with your food; it's like messing with a drug addict by trying to take their substance away. When I'm trying to pull sugar away from you, you tend to get testy, start justifying, or flat out reject the information; but I can tell you that it has major consequences if action is not taken.

Plus, that spare tire around your waist, that stubborn weight that's been around the thighs and in the face and in the neck, that excess weight that you're carrying around is not fat; it's excess sugar. You put in so much excess energy during the day that your body has to come up with a solution as to what to do with it. So, it stores it as fat. Thus, if you want to burn fat, you first have to cut sugar.

Crank UP THE FAT

You need fat to burn fat! Most of the cells in your body are made of fat. Up to 60% of your brain is made of fat. Healthy fat is essential to your health; bad fat is toxic. The low-and no-fat craze hit America over 40 years ago to combat heart disease. What happened? We got fat! Since then, heart disease has skyrocketed. Fat is not the cause of heart disease, sugar is! All that extra weight around your gut is excess sugar that is stored as fat. Sugar can make a good fat/cholesterol turn bad quickly.

If you want to burn up all the fat in your body, one thing must happen nutritionally: you must stop eating sugar. If you do not have sugar as your fuel because you are not eating any of it, then your fuel source becomes fat; you then need to eat fat to spark the engines.

CHALLENGE FOOD GUIDELINES

CLEAN UP THE PROTEIN

This is not a high protein / low carb lifestyle change. Protein is very important, but you don't want too much of it because if you overdo it, it will turn to sugar. Women should eat 15-20 grams per meal and men should eat 20-30 grams per meal. The most important part of protein is to have it clean. Bioaccumulations of toxins are way higher in a non-organic, hormone-loaded 2,000-pound cow than in a head of broccoli. If finances are a concern when it comes to getting healthy food and you find it expensive to eat healthy because of the cost, then focus on the proteins. You'll get the most bang for your buck decreasing toxins when you focus on cleaning up meat and dairy products.

You are not what you eat; you are what you eat, ate.

So, the three main targets for this are beef, chicken, and fish. Pork is out—what does a pig eat? Everything! This makes them very toxic.

A cow is supposed to eat grass. When you feed a cow grain, it gets fat faster, but it makes the cow inflamed and sick. The cow is then pumped full of growth hormones, which makes for more meat, but it starts to get even sicker, so it must be pumped full of antibiotics. Just before it gets too sick to live, it makes it to market and ends up on your plate.

So, cleaning up the beef that you're eating is crucial. Make sure it's organic and grass-fed when possible to eliminate these hormones, the pesticides used in its food, and antibiotics.

When it comes to chicken, we're looking for free- range chicken, not a chicken that's cooped up with 10,000 other chickens standing in their own... well, you know what I'm talking about. Oftentimes, they're fed arsenic in order for them to grow quicker. A chicken in today's world is several times larger than a chicken just 50 or 60 years ago because of all the growth hormones and chemicals that we are adding in to try to make more meat in order to make more profit for the food industry. So, make sure it's organic and free-range when possible to eliminate all those toxic chemicals.

Finally, wild-caught fish: Instead of your salmon or tilapia raised on a farm, confined to a pen, and fed pellets and unnatural foods, you want them free in nature. They then consume what they're designed to consume so that toxins don't end up in you, the top of the food chain.

CHALLENGE FOOD GUIDELINES

C ARE ABOUT NUTRIENTS

It's amazing to me how many children in this country get very little to no nutrients. From whom do you think they learn that? It's amazing to me how many adults in this country get very little to no nutrients.

Throughout the day, a lot can go wrong when it comes to eating right—eat fast food, don't eat at all, eat late. The easiest and most convenient way to take one step toward fixing your food is through breakfast. I believe we have the most opportunity to add health to our lives through breakfast.

The easiest and most convenient way that I found to really alter breakfast is through a breakfast smoothie. In this challenge, I have added several of my favorite smoothie recipes for you. These are go-to smoothie recipes that I use on a regular basis to get nutrients into my body and to keep toxicity out.

In the smoothie, I add lots of veggies like spinach and kale, and then some berries. Putting two huge handfuls of spinach or kale or collard greens into your smoothie is a big way to get a huge dose of nutrients for breakfast. I mean, think about it—when was the last time you had a big bowl of spinach for breakfast? This keeps the sugar down. Then, I add good fat like coconut milk, almond milk, or coconut oil. Finally, I get protein by adding grass-fed whey protein powder. This hits all four C's, fills me up, and energizes me. Make as big of one as you would like!

During the rest of the day drink lots of water and focus on lots of vegetables, greens, and beans—sautéed, baked, steamed, hummus, salads, etc.

My nutrient secret weapon that I suggest is my Livingood Daily Greens which make getting greens quick and easy. It is a simple powder drink that is packed full of nutrients, enzymes, and detoxifiers. This gets nutrients in and also extra water.

Fuel your vehicle, not your cravings.

C URB YOUR CONSUMPTION

If you are struggling to still lose weight and hit health goals after the above four C's of nutrition, then curb your consumption. Take an intermittent fasting approach; this is broken down in your challenge teachings and in the following advanced meal plan.

FOOD LIST

MEATS

- [ ] Beef / Buffalo / Venison
  Ideally All Natural, Best is 100% Grass-Fed & Organic
- [ ] Chicken
  Ideally All Natural, Best is Organic & Free Range
- [ ] Eggs
  Ideally All Natural, Best is Organic & Free Range
- [ ] Fish: Wild Caught

- [ ] Lamb
  Ideally All Natural, Best is 100% Grass-Fed & Organic
- [ ] Turkey
  Ideally All Natural, Best is Organic & Free Range

Avoid
Grain-Fed, Pork, Farm-Raised Fish, Shellfish, and Soy Alternatives

VEGETABLES

[ ] Arugula	[ ] Cucumbers	[ ] Onions	**In Moderation**
[ ] Asparagus	[ ] Dandelion	[ ] Parsley	[ ] Artichokes
[ ] Beans	[ ] Eggplant	[ ] Radishes	[ ] Beets
[ ] Bell Peppers	[ ] Fennel	[ ] Shallots	[ ] Carrots
[ ] Bok Coy	[ ] Garlic	[ ] Snow Peas	[ ] Jicama
[ ] Broccoli	[ ] Green Beans	[ ] Spinach	[ ] Squash
[ ] Brussels Sprouts	[ ] Jalapeno Peppers	[ ] Sprouts	[ ] Sweet Potatoes
[ ] Cabbage	[ ] Kale	[ ] Turnips	[ ] Tomatoes
[ ] Cauliflower	[ ] Kohlrabi	[ ] Water Chestnuts	**Avoid**
[ ] Celery	[ ] Lettuce	[ ] Zucchini	Corn
[ ] Chicory	[ ] Mushrooms		Potatoes
[ ] Collard	[ ] Mustard		

FRUITS

Ideally All Natural, Best is Organic

- [ ] Acai Berries
- [ ] Avocado
- [ ] Blackberries
- [ ] Granny Smith Apples
- [ ] Blueberries

- [ ] Grapefruit
- [ ] Lemon
- [ ] Lime
- [ ] Raspberries
- [ ] Strawberries

Avoid Until Goal Is Hit

[ ] Apricots	[ ] Oranges
[ ] Bananas	[ ] Papaya
[ ] Cherries	[ ] Peaches
[ ] Dates	[ ] Pears
[ ] Grapes	[ ] Pineapple
[ ] Kiwi	[ ] Plum
[ ] Mangoes	[ ] Prunes
[ ] Melon	[ ] Red Apples
[ ] Nectarines	[ ] Dried Fruit
[ ] Watermelon	[ ] Goji Berries

DAIRY

Ideally All Natural, Best is Organic, Full Fat, & Raw - In Moderation

- [ ] Butter
- [ ] Cheese
- [ ] Cream
- [ ] Goat's Milk
- [ ] Goat's Milk Cheese
- [ ] Goat's Milk Yogurt
- [ ] Kefir

- [ ] Organic Milk
- [ ] Almond Milk
- [ ] Cashew Milk
- [ ] Coconut Milk
- [ ] Goat Milk
- [ ] Hemp Milk
- [ ] Ghee

Avoid
Margarine
Shortening
Soy
Non-Organic Dairy

FOOD LIST

NUTS & SEEDS

Best is Raw, Organic and/or Sprouted With No Added Oils
In Moderation

- [ ] Almonds
- [ ] Brazil
- [ ] Cashews
- [ ] Chia Seeds
- [ ] Flax Seeds
- [ ] Hemp Seeds
- [ ] Macadamia

- [ ] Pecans
- [ ] Pine Nuts
- [ ] Pistachios
- [ ] Pumpkin Seeds
- [ ] Sesame Seeds
- [ ] Sunflower Seeds
- [ ] Walnuts

NUT BUTTERS

In Moderation

- [ ] Almond Butter
- [ ] Cashew Butter
- [ ] Macadamia Butter
- [ ] Sunflower Seed Butter
- [ ] Tahini (Raw)

Avoid / Limit

Peanut Butter

OILS

Ideally All Natural, Best is Unrefined & Cold-Pressed

- [ ] Avocado Oil
- [ ] Butter/Ghee (Low Heat)
- [ ] Coconut Oil
- [ ] Flaxseed Oil (Do Not Heat)
- [ ] Grapeseed Oil
- [ ] Olive Oil (Medium/Low Heat)

Avoid

Canola Oil
Corn Oil
Cotton Seed Oil
Rapeseed Oil
Rice Bran Oil
Safflower Oil
Soybean Oil
Sunflower Oil
Vegetable Oil

BEANS

In Moderation

- [ ] Adzuki Beans
- [ ] Black Beans
- [ ] Chickpeas
- [ ] Kidney Beans
- [ ] Legumes

- [ ] Lentils
- [ ] Lima Beans
- [ ] Pinto Beans
- [ ] White Beans

SWEETNERS

- [ ] 100% Stevia
- [ ] Xylitol (In Moderation)
- [ ] Monk Fruit
- [ ] Erythritol

Avoid Until Goal Is Hit
- [ ] Raw Honey
- [ ] Organic Maple Syrup (Grade A/B)

Avoid

All Added Sugars
Aspartame
Dextrose
Fructose
Glucose
Maltodextrin
Splenda
Sucrose

GRAINS

Avoid Until Goal Is Hit

- [ ] Barley
- [ ] Brown/Wild Rice
- [ ] Buckwheat
- [ ] Ezekiel 4:9 Bread
- [ ] Millet
- [ ] Quinoa

- [ ] Rye
- [ ] Spelt
- [ ] Steel Cut Oats
- [ ] Tapioca
- [ ] Sprouted Grain Bread
- [ ] Whole/Wild Grains

BEVERAGES

Best is Unsweetened, Raw or Organic With No Added Sugars | Sweeten with Stevia
In Moderation

- [ ] Coffee
- [ ] Herbal Tea
- [ ] Water (Infused, Purified, And/Or Sparkling)
- [ ] Low Sugar Fruit/Vegetable Juice

Avoid Until Goal Is Hit
- [ ] Fermented Drinks
- [ ] Fruit/Vegetable Juice
- [ ] Coconut Water
- [ ] Zevia/Stevia Sweetened Soda

CONDIMENTS

Best is All Natural or Organic

- [ ] Apple Cider Vinegar
- [ ] Balsamic Vinegar
- [ ] Guacamole
- [ ] Herbs/Spices
- [ ] Hummus (No Bad Oil)
- [ ] Mustard
- [ ] Olive Oil

- [ ] Salsa
- [ ] Sea Salt (Celtic or Himalayan)
- [ ] Soy Sauce (Liquid Aminos, Wheat Free)
- [ ] Mayo (Veganaise or Avocado-Oil Based)

21 DAY MEAL PLAN

WEEK 1

Day			
1	Berry Smoothie	Simple Chicken Salad	Chicken & Broccoli Casserole
2	Egg Scramble	Leftovers	Hamburgers & Zucchini fries
3	Almond Joy Smoothie	Cesar Salad	Chicken Fajitas
4	Egg Bites	Chicken Fajita on Spinach Salad	Meat Stuffed Peppers
5	Berry Smoothie	Leftovers	Chicken Stir-Fry
6	Egg Bites	Leftovers	Shepherd's Pie
7	Smoothie Bowl	Leftovers	Smothered Chicken

WEEK 2

Day			
8	Egg & Turkey Bacon Casserole	Cesar Salad	Baked Chicken & Roasted Brussels
9	Egg & Turkey Bacon Casserole	Leftovers On Salad	Zucchini Spaghetti & Roasted Broccoli
10	Almond Joy Smoothie	Create Your Own Salad	Beef Stir-Fry
11	Fried Eggs & Avocado	You Pick 3	Baked Chicken & Roasted Broccoli
12	Almond Butter Blueberry Smoothie	Leftovers	Chicken & Broccoli Casserole
13	Smoothie Bowl	Leftovers	Enchilada Zucchini Boats
14	Vegetable Omelet	Create Your Own Salad	Vegetable Bean Soup

WEEK 3

Day			
15	Almond Butter Blueberry Smoothie	Leftovers	Hamburgers & Cauliflower Tatoes
16	Turkey Sausage To Go Egg Bakes	You Pick 3	Chili
17	To Go Egg Bakes	Leftovers	Vegetable Stir-Fry
18	Berry Smoothie	Cesar Salad	Steak Fajitas
19	Egg Scramble	Leftovers Over Salad	Meatloaf & Cauliflower Tatoes
20	Smoothie Bowl	Turkey Bacon Cheeseburger Casserole	
21	Vegetable Omelet	Leftovers	Grilled Fish or Meat + Vegetable

Following Week 3, complete a 1, 2, or 3-day liquid fast consuming only water, sparkling water, coffee, tea, Livingood Daily Greens, low-carb greens juice, and/or Livingood Daily Collagen.

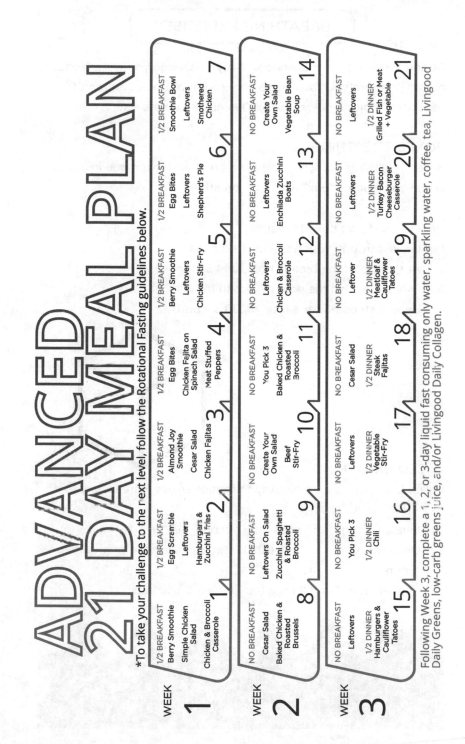

ADVANCED 21 DAY MEAL PLAN

*To take your challenge to the next level, follow the Rotational Fasting guidelines below.

WEEK 1

Day			
1	1/2 BREAKFAST — Berry Smoothie	Simple Chicken Salad	Chicken & Broccoli Casserole
2	1/2 BREAKFAST — Egg Scramble	Leftovers	Hamburgers & Zucchini Fries
3	1/2 BREAKFAST — Almond Joy Smoothie	Cesar Salad	Chicken Fajitas
4	1/2 BREAKFAST — Egg Bites	Chicken Fajita on Spinach Salad	Meat Stuffed Peppers
5	1/2 BREAKFAST — Berry Smoothie	Leftovers	Chicken Stir-Fry
6	1/2 BREAKFAST — Egg Bites	Leftovers	Shepherd's Pie
7	1/2 BREAKFAST — Smoothie Bowl	Leftovers	Smothered Chicken

WEEK 2

Day			
8	NO BREAKFAST	Cesar Salad	Baked Chicken & Roasted Brussels
9	NO BREAKFAST	Leftovers On Salad	Zucchini Spaghetti & Roasted Broccoli
10	NO BREAKFAST	Create Your Own Salad	Beef Stir-Fry
11	NO BREAKFAST	You Pick 3	Baked Chicken & Roasted Broccoli
12	NO BREAKFAST	Leftovers	Chicken & Broccoli Casserole
13	NO BREAKFAST	Leftovers	Enchilada Zucchini Boats
14	NO BREAKFAST	Create Your Own Salad	Vegetable Bean Soup

WEEK 3

Day			
15	NO BREAKFAST	Leftovers	1/2 DINNER — Hamburgers & Cauliflower Tatoes
16	NO BREAKFAST	You Pick 3	1/2 DINNER — Chili
17	NO BREAKFAST	Leftovers	1/2 DINNER — Vegetable Stir-Fry
18	NO BREAKFAST	Cesar Salad	1/2 DINNER — Steak Fajitas
19	NO BREAKFAST	Leftover	1/2 DINNER — Meatloaf & Cauliflower Tatoes
20	NO BREAKFAST	Leftovers	1/2 DINNER — Turkey Bacon Cheeseburger Casserole
21	NO BREAKFAST	Leftovers	1/2 DINNER — Grilled Fish or Meat + Vegetable

Following Week 3, complete a 1, 2, or 3-day liquid fast consuming only water, sparkling water, coffee, tea, Livingood Daily Greens, low-carb greens juice, and/or Livingood Daily Collagen.

BREATHING EXERCISES

During Week 2 of your Livingood Daily Challenge you will introduce breathing exercises. You can do either form of breathing for :60 seconds, 3 times a day, or for 3:00 minutes 1 time a day.

BOXED BREATHING

Boxed breathing is a stress-reducing breathing technique in which you make a "box" with your breath.

Here is how to do boxed breathing:
1. Inhale through your nose for 4 seconds
2. At the top of the breath, hold for 4 seconds
3. Exhale through the nose or mouth for 4 seconds
4. Repeat steps 1-3 for a total of :60 seconds

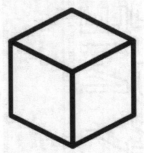

PACED BREATHING

Paced breathing is a simple way to reduce stress. Here is how to do it:
1. Inhale through your nose for 5 seconds
2. Once the lunges are full, exhale through the nose or mouth for 5 seconds
3. Repeat steps 1 and 2 for a total time :60 seconds

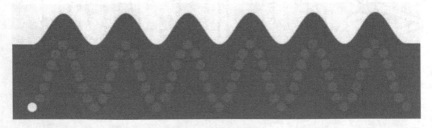

FIX YOUR FRAME

If you wear out the frame and joints of your body there is no replacement and can lead to serious health issues. Each day spend as little as two minutes nurturing and taking care of your posture, joints that need rehabbing, and flexibility. The ideal time is to spend 2 minutes stretching and rehabbing at the end of your 10-minute workout. You can find rehab resources in the online Livingood Daily Challenge or at www.drlivingood.com.

During each day of your challenge, especially starting week 2, add spinal and joint rehab into your routine. This can be done through sleep aids and/or spending 2-10 minutes per day doing posture exercises, rehabbing, and fixing your frame.

CHALLENGE GUIDE

If you focus on building health you will get health. If you focus on your sickness, disease, pills, and problems then all you'll get is more of the same. Each day of your challenge you get the foundational steps to begin building real health. Master the basics of real health and 80% of your problems will go away.

Second, your mind is your super weapon. Each day of your real health journey you are going to use your mind as a secret weapon to drive what you want. In your brain is a center called your reticular activating system (RAS). This works like a google search engine. Whatever you type in it begins to find. If you type in depression, it finds more depression. If you type in joy, it finds joy. If you type in relief, it finds relief. If you type in weight loss, it finds weight loss.

You CAN find whatever health you want in 5 minutes per day. Here is how:

1. Every day write down your goal as if it already achieved. Train your brain that the goal is as good as done.
2. Every day write down everything you are thankful for. Misery is learned. Depression is learned. Anxiety is learned. Gratitude is the anecdote. But it must be learned. Gratitude is like a muscle, it has to be strengthened to be powerful. You can not be stressed and grateful at the same time.
3. Every day keep track of your feedback system. Your body is talking to you. Are you listening? You will be shocked at what you learn by charting how you feel, sleep quality, stress levels, and energy levels each day.
4. Then all you have to do with that information is think about WHY do I feel that way today? What did I or did I not do yesterday that effected my results? Did I eat something poor? Did I lack water? Did I stay up too late? Did I skip my breathing and de-stressing exercises? Did I workout? Did I interact with a negative person or situation? Once you chart your health you can finally see what works best for YOU to experience real health.

Good habits die hard! It takes at least 21 days to create a habit. The only way this doesn't happen is if you get lazy or give up. YOU are more powerful than you think. YOU hold the solution to real health. The greatest doctor in the world is in YOU and YOU have the secret weapon...focus.

I AM THE SOLUTION

- Dr. Livingood

CHALLENGE GUIDE EXAMPLE

Record today's date so you can look back and remember this moment.

DAY 15 | Today's Date _____9/2/19_____

At the end of each day or as you go, check off each thing you accomplished today.

Daily Objectives:

☒ Watched Daily Teaching

☒ Completed 10-Minute Workout + Ab Bonus

☒ No Sugar ☒ 3-6 Servings Healthy Fats & Veggies ☒ Clean Protein

☒ Drank 1/2 My Body Weight In Ounces Of Water

☒ Did My Paced Breathing To De-Stress

☒ 2 Servings of Detoxing Greens

You are 42 percent more likely to achieve your goals if you write them down. Write your goals from your destination page as if they have already happened,

Challenge Goals:

Write your goals for this 21 Day Challenge below as if you have already accomplished them.

I have worked out consistently for the last 21 days!

I have lost 10 lbs and reduced my blood pressure medication!

i have increased my energy and can now play with my kids in the evening!

It's harder to stress or worry when you put your focus on all of the things that are going right for you. Make sure you take time daily to make a note of what you are thankful for.

Today, I'm Grateful For:

Getting to eat breakfast together as a family this morning.

Health Tracker:

Use this space to track anything health related during your journey so you can see progress. To Live Good Daily is to realize this is a journey and not a temporary fix.

For Example:

My Blood Pressure: 130/86

Stress Level 1-10: 4

Sleep Quality 1-10: 8

Energy Level 1-10: 8

*I've noticed that working out in the morning has lowered my stress/anxiety level while at work

Today I Feel:

I Feel This Way Because:

Got up on 1st alarm

Coffee date with Zach

But stressed with big

deadline at work

DAY 1 | Today's Date _____

Daily Objectives:

- O Watched Daily Teaching
- O Completed 10-Minute Workout + Ab Bonus
- O No Sugar   O 3-6 Servings Healthy Fats & Veggies   O Clean Protein
- O Drank 1/2 My Body Weight In Ounces Of Water

Challenge Goals:
Write your goals for this 21 Day Challenge below as if you have already accomplished them.

_____

_____

_____

_____

_____

Today, I'm Grateful For:

_____

_____

Health Tracker:

Today I Feel:

☹ ☹ 😐 🙂 😄
– [========] +

I Feel This Way Because:

_____

_____

_____

_____

Berry Smoothie

Serves 1 | 10 Minutes

2 handfuls of spinach
and/or kale

1/4-1/2 can of full-fat
coconut milk

1/2 cup of water

1-2 cups of frozen berries
(if using fresh berries add
3-4 ice cubes)

1 scoop Livingood Daily
Collagen Protein Vanilla

Combine all ingredients in a
high-powered blender and mix.
Use more or less of any ingredient
to make thicker, thinner, or colder.

Simple Chicken Salad

Serves 2 | 30 Minutes

Combine all ingredients in a bowl.
Can also add things like avocado,
dried cranberries, grapes, or raisins,
if desired (watch if on a low/no
sugar based plan). Serve over a bed
of spinach or on romaine
lettuce wraps.

2 cooked chicken
breasts

1 cup celery, diced

1/4 cup chopped
walnuts or slivered
almonds

2 tsp lemon juice or
apple cider vinegar

2/3 cup Vegenaise (no
soy) (or use a healthy oil
mayo)

Salt and pepper, to taste

Chicken & Broccoli Casserole

Serves 4 | 45 Minutes

3 chicken breasts

2 bunches of broccoli

8 oz organic shredded cheddar cheese

1 bunch green onion, 4-5 sliced

Salt, pepper, garlic powder (to taste)

2 tbsp multipurpose seasoning (watch ingredients)

1 1/2 cups sliced almonds

1/2 stick organic butter

1/2 cup Vegenaise (or healthy oil based mayo)

Boil chicken until tender. Season and cut into cubes. Steam broccoli until tender. Combine all ingredients except almonds and butter and mix well. Press into a 9x13 baking dish. Sprinkle with almonds on top and drizzle with melted butter. Bake at 375 degrees for approximately 30 minutes.

DAY 2 | Today's Date _____

Daily Objectives:

- O Watched Daily Teaching
- O Completed 10-Minute Workout + Ab Bonus
- O No Sugar   O 3-6 Servings Healthy Fats & Veggies   O Clean Protein
- O Drank 1/2 My Body Weight In Ounces Of Water

Challenge Goals:
Write your goals for this 21 Day Challenge below as if you have already accomplished them.

_____

_____

_____

_____

_____

Today, I'm Grateful For:

_____

_____

_____

Health Tracker:

Today I Feel:

☹ ☹ 😐 🙂 😄

− ▭▭▭▭▭ +

I Feel This Way Because:

_____

_____

_____

_____

Egg Scramble

Serves 1 | 20 Minutes

2 eggs

1/2 cup vegetables (bell peppers, spinach, zucchini, mushrooms, broccoli, onion, etc)

1/2 cup turkey bacon or turkey sausage, cooked (optional)

Salt, pepper (to taste)

2 tbsp coconut oil

Optional toppings: avocado, cheese, (cheddar, feta, goat, etc), chives

Whisk eggs, veggies, pre-cooked meat, and seasonings in a bowl. In a medium pan, heat oil over medium-low heat. Cook 6-8 minutes until eggs are cooked through. Top with favorite toppings.

Vegetarian Plan Tip: Approved for vegetarians that eat eggs and/or dairy. Avoid turkey bacon/sausage and sautee another 1/2 cup of veggies of your choice if you desire.

Hamburgers

Serves 2 | 30 Minutes

Grill, or cook slowly in coconut oil, hamburger patties with seasoning until preferred temperature. Wrap in romaine lettuce leaves and top with preferred toppings. Cook extra to use as leftover hamburger for lunch or to create a salad the next day.

Vegetarian Plan Tip:
Opt for a black bean burger. Heat the olive oil in a skillet over medium-high heat. Saute the onion until soft, about 5 minutes, then add in the garlic and stir for one more minute. Remove from the heat. In a large bowl, combine the sauteed onion and garlic, beans, sweet potato, ground flax, cumin and salt. Use a fork to stir the mixture, mashing the beans to help the batter stick together. Scoop out the black bean mixture and use your hands to shape it into a burger about 3/4-inch thick. Line a baking sheet with parchment paper. Bake the burgers at 350F for 15 minutes, then use a spatula to gently flip them over and bake for another 5 to 10 minutes.

1 lb grass-fed beef

Salt, pepper, garlic salt (to taste)

Romaine lettuce leaves

Optional Toppings: ketchup, organic cheese, mustard, pickles, onions, avocado, turkey bacon, fried egg, etc

Black Bean Burger (Optional):
2 (15 oz.) cans black beans , drained and rinsed

1 tbsp olive oil

1/2 yellow onion , chopped

3 cloves garlic , minced

1/2 cup mashed sweet potato (steamed, then mashed)

1/4 cup ground flax seeds

1/2 tsp ground cumin

1/2 tsp salt

Zucchini Fries

Serves 2 | 30 Minutes

1 large organic zucchini

1 cup almond flour

Salt, pepper, garlic powder (or any cajun or multi purpose spice, check ingredients)

2 eggs, beaten

Combine almond flour and seasoning in a small bowl. Cut zucchini into fry-sized rectangles. Dip zucchini in egg and then dip and cover in flour mixture. Bake on parchment lined baking sheet at 425 degrees for 20-30 minutes or until brown and crispy.

Vegetarian Plan Tip: Approved for vegetarians that eat eggs and/or dairy.

DAY 3 | Today's Date _____

Daily Objectives:

O Watched Daily Teaching

O Completed 10-Minute Workout + Ab Bonus

O No Sugar   O 3-6 Servings Healthy Fats & Veggies   O Clean Protein

O Drank 1/2 My Body Weight In Ounces Of Water

Challenge Goals:
Write your goals for this 21 Day Challenge below as if you have already accomplished them.

_____

_____

_____

_____

_____

Today, I'm Grateful For:

_____

_____

_____

Health Tracker:

Today I Feel:

– ⬚⬚⬚⬚⬚ +

I Feel This Way Because:

_____

_____

_____

_____

Almond Joy Smoothie

Serves 1 | 5 Minutes

1 scoop Livingood
Daily Collagen Protein
Chocolate (or 1 tbsp
cocoa powder)

2 tbsp raw almond or
nut butter

1 tsp cinnamon

1 tsp pure vanilla
extract

1 cup unsweetened
almond milk or full-fat
coconut milk

1/2 a frozen avocado or
banana (optional)

3-4 ice cubes
(optional)

Put all ingredients in a blender and
mix. Can add more or less milk and
ice depending consistency and
temperature desired.

Cesar Salad

Serves 2 | 20 Minutes

Mix or blend all dressing ingredients together until smooth. Combine chicken, spinach, romaine, and dressing in a bowl with a lid and shake until completely covered. Add more parmesan cheese to the top before eating.

Vegetarian Plan Tip:
Approved for vegetarians that eat eggs and/or dairy. Simply leave off cooked chicken.

2 chicken breasts, cooked how desired

Organic spinach and romaine lettuce

Dressing:
1/2 cup olive oil

1 lemon (juiced, can add zest as well)

1/3 cup parmesan cheese

4 tsp dijon mustard (no sugar)

1-2 garlic cloves or garlic powder

Worcestershire sauce, to taste (no sugar)

Salt and pepper, to taste

Chicken Fajitas

Serves 2 | 25 Minutes

2 tbsp coconut oil

2 organic chicken breasts

1 small red onion, sliced

1 organic red bell peppers, sliced

1 organic green bell pepper, sliced (or any color bell pepper)

Spinach or romaine lettuce

Seasoning: 2 tbsp chili powder, 3 tbsp cumin, salt, pepper, garlic powder

Optional Toppings: raw organic cheddar cheese, black beans, organic sour cream, cilantro, cucumber, avocado, salsa

Saute chicken in coconut oil over medium heat until cooked entirely. Add vegetables and seasoning (may add a little water to help steam the vegetables). Cook until vegetables are tender. Put on a plate of spinach and top with desired toppings.

Vegetarian Plan Tip: Replace meat with 2 cups of veggies of your choice from the Food List.

DAY 4 | Today's Date _____

Daily Objectives:

O Watched Daily Teaching

O Completed 10-Minute Workout + Ab Bonus

O No Sugar   O 3-6 Servings Healthy Fats & Veggies   O Clean Protein

O Drank 1/2 My Body Weight In Ounces Of Water

Challenge Goals:
Write your goals for this 21 Day Challenge below as if you have already accomplished them.

_____

_____

_____

_____

_____

Today, I'm Grateful For:

_____

_____

_____

Health Tracker:

Today I Feel:

– ☹ ☹ 😐 🙂 😄 +

I Feel This Way Because:

_____

_____

_____

_____

Egg Bites

Yields 6 Muffins | 30 Minutes

8 eggs

1 cup vegetables - diced
(ex: broccoli, bell
peppers, onion,
mushrooms, etc)

1/4 cup almond milk

Salt & pepper (to taste)
(or any other seasoning)

1/2 cup raw or organic
cheese (optional)

1/2 cup turkey bacon,
cooked (optional)

1 tbsp coconut oil

Lightly grease muffin tin with
coconut oil. Whisk all ingredients
together. Pour into muffin tins.
Bake 350 degrees F for 20-25
minutes.

Vegetarian Plan Tip:
Approved for vegetarians that eat
eggs and/or dairy.

Meat Stuffed Peppers
Serves 4 | 60 Minutes

Preheat oven to 400 degrees F. Sauté meat and onions over low/medium heat in pan until browned. Meanwhile, place peppers cut side down on baking sheet and bake until tender, approximately 20–25 minutes.

Stir meat and onion, seasoning, aminos, and tomato sauce. Fill pepper halves mixture. Bake 5-10 minutes or until heated through. Can top with Parmesan or any cheese if desired. Can serve with Mashed Cauliflower Tatoes or steamed vegetables.

*Can also add 1/2 cup cooked quinoa if desired and not on a low carb plan.

Vegetarian Plan Tip:
Substitute ground beef with 1 bag of cauliflower rice (or 1 head of cauliflower, riced) and reduce cook time by a couple minutes.

4 red, green, yellow, or orange bell peppers

1.5 pounds grass-fed ground beef

1 small onion, diced

1 small can organic, Italian-style diced tomatoes

2 tbsp Braggs Liquid Aminos

Salt, pepper, garlic

OFFICIALLY OFF OF HER BLOOD PRESSURE AND CHOLESTEROL MEDICATIONS AND LOST 10 POUNDS!

OFF OF ALL MEDICATIONS & LOST 50LBS!

BLOOD PRESSURE, CHOLESTEROL IMPROVING & NO LONGER HAS VERTIGO IN JUST 3 MONTHS!

DAY 5 | Today's Date _____

Daily Objectives:

- O Watched Daily Teaching
- O Completed 10-Minute Workout + Ab Bonus
- O No Sugar   O 3-6 Servings Healthy Fats & Veggies   O Clean Protein
- O Drank 1/2 My Body Weight In Ounces Of Water

Challenge Goals:
Write your goals for this 21 Day Challenge below as if you have already accomplished them.

_____

_____

_____

_____

_____

Today, I'm Grateful For:

_____

_____

_____

Health Tracker:

Today I Feel:

Today I Feel:

I Feel This Way Because:

_____

_____

_____

_____

Berry Smoothie

Serves 1 | 10 Minutes

2 handfuls of spinach
and/or kale

1/4-1/2 can of full-fat
coconut milk

1/2 cup of water

1-2 cups of frozen berries
(if using fresh berries add
3-4 ice cubes)

1 scoop Livingood Daily
Collagen Protein Vanilla

Combine all ingredients in a
high-powered blender and mix. Use
more or less of any ingredient to make
thicker, thinner, or colder.

Chicken Stir Fry

Serves 2 | 20 Minutes

Sauté chicken in coconut oil until cooked. Add vegetables and seasonings and sauté until tender. Can serve over cauliflower rice if preferred.

Vegetarian Plan Tip:
Replace meat with 2 cups of veggies of your choice from the Food List.

4 tbsp coconut oil

2 chicken breasts, cut into bite-sized pieces

Variety of vegetables: broccoli, bell peppers, onion, snap peas, zucchini, squash, peas, cauliflower, mushrooms, carrots, etc. (as many as desired)

Salt, pepper, garlic powder (to taste)

3 tbsp Braggs Liquid Aminos (more or less to taste)

NO MORE PAIN, MEMORY IMPROVED!

PAMELA IS HEART MED AND DIABETES MED FREE AFTER JUST 6 WEEKS!

CUT THYROID MEDICATIONS IN HALF & LOST 10.5 LBS IN THE WEIGHT LOSS HEALTH POTENTIAL CHURCH CHALLENGE!

OUT OF PAIN AND NO MORE HANDICAP STICKER NEEDED!

DAY 6 | Today's Date _____

Daily Objectives:

- O Watched Daily Teaching

- O Completed 10-Minute Workout + Ab Bonus

- O No Sugar   O 3-6 Servings Healthy Fats & Veggies   O Clean Protein

- O Drank 1/2 My Body Weight In Ounces Of Water

Challenge Goals:
Write your goals for this 21 Day Challenge below as if you have already
accomplished them.

_____

_____

_____

_____

_____

Today, I'm Grateful For:

_____

_____

_____

Health Tracker:

Today I Feel:

– +

I Feel This Way Because:

_____

_____

_____

_____

Egg Bites

Yields 6 Muffins | 30 Minutes

8 eggs

1 cup vegetables – diced
(ex: broccoli, bell
peppers, onion,
mushrooms, etc)

1/4 cup almond milk

Salt & pepper (to taste)
(or any other seasoning)

1/2 cup raw or organic
cheese (optional)

1/2 cup turkey bacon,
cooked (optional)

1 tbsp coconut oil

Lightly grease muffin tin with
coconut oil. Whisk all ingredients
together. Pour into muffin tins.
Bake 350 degrees F for 20-25
minutes.

Vegetarian Plan Tip:
Approved for vegetarians that eat
eggs and/or dairy.

Shepherd's Pie
Serves 4 | 60 Minutes

Brown hamburger, add in onion, carrots, peas and let steam until tender, approximately 10 minutes. In separate saucepan, simmer beef broth and cauliflower rice for approximately 10 minutes. Remove from heat and add seasonings, Worcestershire sauce, and butter. Put all ingredients into a blender and mix until smooth, adding in the arrowroot powder until it becomes a puree. Pour over the meat and vegetables in an 8×8 baking dish and top with mashed cauliflower tatoes. Bake at 350 degrees F until warm throughout or until top starts to brown.

Topping:
Mashed Cauliflower Tatoes Recipe
1 head cauliflower
Salt and pepper, to taste
4 tbs organic butter
Garlic powder (optional)
Steam cauliflower in steamer until tender. In blender mix cauliflower, butter and seasonings until smooth.

Inside:
1 lb grass-fed ground beef
1/2 small onion, diced
3 carrots, diced
1 cup peas

Sauce:
4 tbsp butter
2 cups beef bone broth
1/2 small onion, diced
1 cup cauliflower rice
Salt and pepper, to taste
Garlic powder, to taste
2 tsp Worcestershire sauce
1/2 cup arrowroot powder

CINDY LOST 20LBS IN JUST 21 DAYS!

OFF SLEEP MEDICATIONS, ANTIDEPRESSANTS & ACID REFLUX MEDICATIONS AND DOWN 21 POUNDS!

OFF BLOOD PRESSURE MEDICATION, NO BACK PAIN, LOST 15LBS.

DAY 7 | Today's Date _____

Daily Objectives:

- O Watched Daily Teaching
- O Completed 10-Minute Workout + Ab Bonus
- O No Sugar   O 3-6 Servings Healthy Fats & Veggies   O Clean Protein
- O Drank 1/2 My Body Weight In Ounces Of Water

Challenge Goals:
Write your goals for this 21 Day Challenge below as if you have already accomplished them.

_____

_____

_____

_____

_____

Today, I'm Grateful For:

_____

_____

_____

Health Tracker:

Today I Feel:

Today I Feel:

I Feel This Way Because:

_____

_____

_____

_____

Smoothie Bowl
Serves 1 | 15 Minutes

1/2-1 cup coconut or almond milk

1 1/2 cup frozen berries of choice (acai, blueberries, blackberries, strawberries, raspberries, etc. - can add 1/2 fresh or frozen banana for thicker consistency)

1/2 scoop Livingood Daily Collagen Protein Vanilla (optional)

Ice to thicken consistency, if desired

Optional Toppings: sliced fruit or berries, coconut flakes, chia seeds, cacao nibs or 70% or greater stevia sweetened dark chocolate chips

Put all ingredients in a high-powered blender or food processor and blend until thick, smoothie-like consistency. Add more ice or berries if you prefer thicker bowls. Pour the smoothie bowl mixture into a bowl and top with your favorite toppings! Enjoy immediately!

Smothered Chicken
Serves 2 | 45 Minutes

Bake seasoned chicken at 350 degrees F in small baking dish until cooked through, approximately 45 minutes. Saute veggies in coconut oil in frying pan. Place the sauteed veggies on top of the chicken once done. Cover with black beans. Top with cheese. Place back in the oven to melt the cheese. Top with optional toppings and salsa.

We like to smother a whole chicken breast with the ingredients. You may also chop up the chicken and serve on top of a salad.

Vegetarian Plan Tip:
Approved for vegetarians that eat eggs and/or dairy. Simply remove chicken or sautee cauliflower florets with the same seasonings.

2 chicken breasts

3 tbsp coconut oil

1 green bell pepper, sliced

1 red bell pepper, sliced

1 small red onion, sliced

1 can black beans

1 cup raw or organic cheddar cheese, shredded

2 tbsp salsa (check ingredients)

Salt, pepper, cumin, garlic powder, chili powder (to taste)

LESS NUMBNESS & TINGLING, NO LOW BACK PAIN OR SLEEP ISSUES AND LOST 15 POUNDS!

NO MORE BLADDER PROBLEMS OR DEPRESSION!

NO MORE SNORING, NO ALLERGIES, NO MORE HEADACHES!

DAY 8 | Today's Date _____

Daily Objectives:

- O Watched Daily Teaching
- O Completed 10-Minute Workout + Ab Bonus
- O No Sugar   O 3-6 Servings Healthy Fats & Veggies   O Clean Protein
- O Drank 1/2 My Body Weight In Ounces Of Water
- O Did My Paced Breathing To De-Stress

Challenge Goals:
Write your goals for this 21 Day Challenge below as if you have already accomplished them.

_____

_____

_____

_____

_____

Today, I'm Grateful For:

_____

_____

_____

Health Tracker:

Today I Feel:

– 😞 😟 😐 😊 😄 +

I Feel This Way Because:

_____

_____

_____

Egg & Turkey Bacon Casserole

Serves 4 | 40 Minutes

8 organic eggs

8 oz organic turkey bacon or 1/2 pound turkey sausage

1 cup coconut milk or unsweetened almond milk

1 1/2 cups organic shredded cheddar cheese

Salt and pepper, to taste

Any herb of choice for topping (optional)

Optional: vegetables such as onion, spinach, bell peppers, mushrooms, etc.

Cook meat in a frying pan until cooked through. Beat eggs and milk together and add cooked meat, half of the cheese, and seasoning. Sprinkle the remaining cheese on top. Using organic butter or coconut oil grease the bottom of an 8×8 baking dish. Bake at 350 degrees F for approximately 20-30 minutes until golden brown.

Vegetarian Plan Tip:
Approved for vegetarians that eat eggs and/or dairy. Avoid turkey bacon/sausage and sautee another 1/2 cup of veggies of your choice if you desire.

Cesar Salad
Serves 2 | 20 Minutes

Mix or blend all dressing ingredients together until smooth. Combine chicken, spinach, romaine, and dressing in a bowl with a lid and shake until completely covered. Add more parmesan cheese to the top before eating.

Vegetarian Plan Tip:
Approved for vegetarians that eat eggs and/or dairy. Simply remove cooked chicken.

2 chicken breasts, cooked how desired

Organic spinach and romaine lettuce

Dressing:
1/2 cup olive oil

1 lemon (juiced, can add zest as well)

1/3 cup parmesan cheese

4 tsp dijon mustard (no sugar)

1-2 garlic cloves or garlic powder

Worcestershire sauce, to taste (no sugar)

Salt and pepper, to taste

Baked Chicken & Roasted Brussels

Serves 2 | 40 Minutes

Chicken:
2 chicken breasts

Salt, pepper, garlic powder (to taste)

Teriyaki Sauce (Coconut Secret brand Teriyaki Sauce - optional)

Roasted Brussels:
1 bag of fresh or frozen sprouts (if fresh, cut end off and cut in half)

3 tbsp olive oil or avocado oil

Salt and pepper (to taste)

Garlic powder (to taste)

Optional toppings: parmesan cheese or balsamic vinegar

Bake chicken in a small baking dish at 350 degrees F with seasonings or sauce desired for approximately 40 minutes or until cooked through (cover with foil). Can put 1-2 tbsp water or butter in dish for moisture. Can make extra and use as leftovers for lunch or to create a salad with. Serve over cauliflower rice if desired.

Toss the brussels sprouts with oil and seasoning. Spread them out and bake at 425 degrees F until tender and outsides are starting to brown. Approximately 30 minutes. Can broil them at the end if want more crisp.

Vegetarian Plan Tip:
Substitute chicken for 2 cups of sauteed cauliflower florets.

DAY 9 | Today's Date _____

Daily Objectives:

- O Watched Daily Teaching
- O Completed 10-Minute Workout + Ab Bonus
- O No Sugar   O 3-6 Servings Healthy Fats & Veggies   O Clean Protein
- O Drank 1/2 My Body Weight In Ounces Of Water
- O Did My Paced Breathing To De-Stress

Challenge Goals:
Write your goals for this 21 Day Challenge below as if you have already accomplished them.

_____

_____

_____

_____

_____

Today, I'm Grateful For:

_____

_____

_____

Health Tracker:

Today I Feel:

😦 😟 😐 🙂 😄
− ▢▭▭▭▭▭ +

I Feel This Way Because:

_____

_____

_____

_____

Egg & Turkey Bacon Casserole

Serves 4 | 40 Minutes

8 organic eggs

8 oz organic turkey bacon or 1/2 pound turkey sausage

1 cup coconut milk or unsweetened almond milk

1 1/2 cups organic shredded cheddar cheese

Salt and pepper, to taste

Any herb of choice for topping (optional)

Optional: vegetables such as onion, spinach, bell peppers, mushrooms, etc.

Cook meat in a frying pan until cooked through. Beat eggs and milk together and add cooked meat, half of the cheese, and seasoning. Sprinkle the remaining cheese on top. Using organic butter or coconut oil grease the bottom of an 8×8 baking dish. Bake at 350 degrees F for approximately 20-30 minutes until golden brown.

Vegetarian Plan Tip: Approved for vegetarians that eat eggs and/or dairy. Avoid turkey bacon/sausage and sautee another 1/2 cup of veggies of your choice if you desire.

Zucchini Spaghetti

Serves 2 | 25 Minutes

In a large pan, brown hamburger and season with salt and pepper. Once the hamburger is cooked through, add the sauce into the pan If making your own sauce, you can put all sauce ingredients right into the pan with the hamburger, stir and warm. Mix the zucchini noodles into the sauce mix. If you are spiralizing your own noodles, simply follow the tool's instructions. You may need to press the noodles down a bit to submerge the sauce. Simmer for approximately 10 minutes or until noodles are tender.

Vegetarian Plan Tip:
Simply remove ground beef.

1 lb grass-fed beef

2 zucchini (cut into long thin strands, use a spiralizer, or buy pre-spiralized noodles)

1 jar spaghetti sauce (or make your own, see below)

Spaghetti Sauce:
1 can organic tomato sauce
1 can organic diced tomatoes
1 6oz can of organic tomato paste
1 tsp dried basil
1/2 tsp dried oregano
1/2 tsp garlic powder
1/2 tsp onion powder
1/4 tsp ground thyme
Salt and pepper, to taste

Roasted Broccoli

Serves 2 | 30 Minutes

2 large heads of broccoli

3 tbsp olive oil or avocado oil

Salt and pepper, to taste

Garlic salt (optional)

Parmesan cheese (optional)

Toss the broccoli florets with oil and seasoning. Spread them out and roast on 425 degrees F until the edges are crispy and the stems are tender. Approximately 30 minutes. Can broil them at the end if want more crisp. Can also top with parmesan cheese when done cooking.

DAY 10 | Today's Date _____

Daily Objectives:

- O Watched Daily Teaching
- O Completed 10-Minute Workout + Ab Bonus
- O No Sugar   O 3-6 Servings Healthy Fats & Veggies   O Clean Protein
- O Drank 1/2 My Body Weight In Ounces Of Water
- O Did My Paced Breathing To De-Stress

Challenge Goals:
Write your goals for this 21 Day Challenge below as if you have already accomplished them.

_____

_____

_____

_____

_____

Today, I'm Grateful For:

_____

_____

_____

Health Tracker:

Today I Feel:

☹ ☹ 😐 🙂 😊

– ▭▭▭▭▭ +

I Feel This Way Because:

_____

_____

_____

_____

Almond Joy Smoothie

Serves 1 | 5 Minutes

1 scoop Livingood Daily Collagen Protein Chocolate (or 1 tbsp cocoa powder)

2 tbsp raw almond or nut butter

1 tsp cinnamon

1 tsp pure vanilla extract

1/4-1/2 can unsweetened almond milk or full-fat coconut milk

1/2 a frozen avocado or banana (optional)

3-4 ice cubes (optional)

Put all ingredients in a blender and mix. Can add more or less milk and ice depending consistency and temperature desired.

Create Your Own Salad

May we suggest putting together a creation of choice. Here are a few ideas...

Mediterranean Style: chicken, cucumbers, feta cheese, red onion, kalamata olives

Simple Salad: meat or fish, any vegetables left over in your fridge, hard-boiled egg

Sweet & Nutty: meat of choice, berries, nuts, gorgonzola or goat cheese

Beef Stir Fry

Serves 2 | 30 Minutes

3 tbsp coconut oil

1 lb grass-fed beef

Salt, pepper, garlic powder (to taste)

3 tbsp Braggs Liquid Aminos (more or less to taste)

Variety of vegetables: broccoli, bell peppers, onion, snap peas, zucchini, squash, mushrooms, peas, cauliflower, carrots, etc.

Brown hamburger in coconut oil until cooked. Add vegetables and seasonings and sauté until tender. Can serve over cauliflower rice or add in cooked rice noodles if preferred.

Vegetarian Plan Tip: Replace meat with 2 cups of diced veggies of your choice from the Food List.

DAY 11 | Today's Date _____

Daily Objectives:

- O Watched Daily Teaching

- O Completed 10-Minute Workout + Ab Bonus

- O No Sugar   O 3-6 Servings Healthy Fats & Veggies   O Clean Protein

- O Drank 1/2 My Body Weight In Ounces Of Water

- O Did My Paced Breathing To De-Stress

Challenge Goals:
Write your goals for this 21 Day Challenge below as if you have already accomplished them.

_____

_____

_____

_____

_____

Today, I'm Grateful For:

_____

_____

_____

Health Tracker:

Today I Feel:

☹ 🙁 😐 🙂 😊

− ▭▭▭▭▭▭▭ +

I Feel This Way Because:

_____

_____

_____

_____

Fried Eggs & Avocado
Serves 2 | 5 Minutes

2 eggs

Salt and pepper, to taste

2 tbsp coconut oil

Melt coconut oil in a frying pan on medium-low heat. Once melted, add the two eggs. Cook until the eggs are cooked on one side, approximately 3-4 minutes. Flip the eggs gently with a spatula and cook another 2-3 minutes depending on how you like your eggs. Salt, pepper, chives on top and enjoy! Add some avocado on the side for some good fats!

Vegetarian Plan Tip:
Approved for vegetarians that eat eggs and/or dairy.

You Pick 3

Pick a few of the following items and have a lighter "grazing" lunch! Find your own items to add to your list!

Hard-boiled eggs

Raw veggies & guacamole

Raw veggies & hummus

Turkey & hummus roll ups

Raw organic cheese chunks

Olives

Berries

Apple slices with almond butter

Nuts

Side salad with leftover meat and veggies

Pickles

Smoothie

Baked Chicken & Roasted Broccoli

Serves 2 | 40 Minutes

2 chicken breasts

Salt, pepper, garlic powder (to taste)

Teriyaki Sauce
(Coconut Secret brand Teriyaki Sauce)
(optional)

2 large heads of broccoli

3 tbsp olive oil or avocado oil

Salt and pepper, to taste
Garlic salt (optional)

Parmesan cheese (optional)

Bake chicken in a small baking dish at 350 degrees F with seasonings or sauce desired for approximately 40 minutes or until cooked through (cover with foil). Can put 1-2 tbsp water or butter in dish for moisture. Can make extra and use as leftovers for lunch or to create a salad with. Serve over cauliflower rice if desired.

Toss the broccoli florets with oil and seasoning. Spread them out and roast on 425 degrees F until the edges are crispy and the stems are tender. Approximately 30 minutes. Can broil them at the end if want more crisp. Can also top with parmesan cheese when done cooking.

Vegetarian Plan Tip:
Replace meat with 2 cups of veggies of your choice from the Food List.

DAY 12 | Today's Date _____

Daily Objectives:

- O Watched Daily Teaching
- O Completed 10-Minute Workout + Ab Bonus
- O No Sugar   O 3-6 Servings Healthy Fats & Veggies   O Clean Protein
- O Drank 1/2 My Body Weight In Ounces Of Water
- O Did My Paced Breathing To De-Stress

Challenge Goals:
Write your goals for this 21 Day Challenge below as if you have already accomplished them.

_____

_____

_____

_____

_____

Today, I'm Grateful For:

_____

_____

_____

Health Tracker:

Today I Feel:

– ☹ 🙁 😐 🙂 😊 +

I Feel This Way Because:

_____

_____

_____

_____

Almond Butter Blueberry Smoothie

Serves 1 | 10 Minutes

1 large handful of
spinach

1/4-1/2 can full-fat
coconut milk and/or
unsweetened vanilla
almond milk

1/2 -1 cup frozen
blueberries

1 heaping spoonful raw
almond butter

1 scoop Livingood Daily
Collagen Protein Vanilla

1 tsp Cacao nibs
(optional)

1 tsp Flax and/or chia
seeds (optional)

Ice (3-4 pieces)

Blend all ingredients in a blender
until smooth. Add more milk as
needed depending on desired
consistency.

Chicken & Broccoli Casserole
Serves 4 | 45 Minutes

Boil chicken until tender. Season and cut into cubes. Steam broccoli until tender. Combine all ingredients except almonds and butter and mix well. Press into a 9x13 baking dish. Sprinkle with almonds on top and drizzle with melted butter. Bake at 375 degrees for approximately 30 minutes.

3 chicken breasts

2 bunches of broccoli

8 oz organic shredded cheddar cheese

1 bunch green onion, 4-5 sliced

Salt, pepper, garlic powder (to taste)

2 tbsp multipurpose seasoning (watch ingredients)

1 1/2 cups sliced almonds

1/2 stick organic butter

1/2 cup Vegenaise (or healthy oil based mayo)

OFF OF ALL MIGRAINE MEDICATIONS!

PATIENT OF 4 YEARS IS STILL ACHE-FREE!

FAMILY OF 6 HAVE BEEN LIVING A DRUG FREE LIFESTYLE FOR 6 YEARS!

THIRD GENERATION OF HER FAMILY TO BE A PATIENT HERE IN THE CLINIC! Her mom has better digestions & headaches are gone and dad is correcting his scoliosis!

DAY 13 | Today's Date _____

Daily Objectives:

O Watched Daily Teaching

O Completed 10-Minute Workout + Ab Bonus

O No Sugar   O 3-6 Servings Healthy Fats & Veggies   O Clean Protein

O Drank 1/2 My Body Weight In Ounces Of Water

O Did My Paced Breathing To De-Stress

Challenge Goals:
Write your goals for this 21 Day Challenge below as if you have already accomplished them.

_____

_____

_____

_____

_____

Today, I'm Grateful For:

_____

_____

_____

Health Tracker:

Today I Feel:

$-$ +

I Feel This Way Because:

_____

_____

_____

_____

215

Smoothie Bowl

Serves 1 | 15 Minutes

1/2-1 cup coconut or almond milk

1 1/2 cup frozen berries of choice (acai, blueberries, blackberries, strawberries, raspberries, etc. - can add 1/2 fresh or frozen banana for thicker consistency)

1/2 scoop Livingood Daily Collagen Protein Vanilla (optional)

Ice to thicken consistency, if desired

Optional Toppings: sliced fruit or berries, coconut flakes, chia seeds, cacao nibs or 70% or greater stevia sweetened dark chocolate chips

Put all ingredients in a high-powered blender or food processor and blend until thick, smoothie-like consistency. Add more ice or berries if you prefer thicker bowls. Pour the smoothie bowl mixture into a bowl and top with your favorite toppings! Enjoy immediately!

Enchilada Zucchini Boats
Serves 2 | 35 Minutes

Cut zucchini in half the long way and gently scoop out most of the inside of the zucchini. In a frying pan, warm the oil and add the seasonings, onion and pepper to saute until soft. Add in the black beans and cook another 3 minutes. Place the zucchini in a lightly greased baking dish, spoon the enchilada mix into the zucchinis, and top them with enchilada sauce, Top with cheese and bake for approximately 25-30 minutes at 400 degrees F.

1 tablespoon of oil

1/2 of a sweet onion

1/2 red bell pepper

3 cloves of garlic, minced (or ½ tsp garlic powder)

1/4 teaspoon of cumin

1/4 teaspoon of dried oregano

1/4 teaspoon of paprika

Sea salt and pepper, to taste

1 can of black beans, drained

2 medium zucchinis

1 1/2 cups of enchilada sauce (watch ingredients on the package)

Optional toppings: organic cheese, cilantro, sour cream

10 YEARS WITH SEVERE ALLERGIES & MIGRAINES GONE!

WELCOME TO THE WORLD, BABY MILAN! Keeping kids healthy from birth!

AVOIDED BACK SURGERY AT AGE 15, NO MORE PAIN AND BETTER SLEEP!

SLEEPING WITHOUT TAKING AMBIEN!

DAY 14 | Today's Date _____

Daily Objectives:

O Watched Daily Teaching

O Completed 10-Minute Workout + Ab Bonus

O No Sugar   O 3-6 Servings Healthy Fats & Veggies   O Clean Protein

O Drank 1/2 My Body Weight In Ounces Of Water

O Did My Paced Breathing To De-Stress

Challenge Goals:
Write your goals for this 21 Day Challenge below as if you have already accomplished them.

_____

_____

_____

_____

_____

Today, I'm Grateful For:

_____

_____

_____

Health Tracker:

Today I Feel:

– ☹ ☹ 😐 🙂 😀 +

I Feel This Way Because:

_____

_____

_____

_____

Vegetable Omelet
Serves 1 | 15 Minutes

3 eggs

1 cup vegetables (bell peppers, spinach, onion, broccoli, mushrooms, asparagus, etc)

Salt, pepper (to taste)

2 tbsp coconut oil

1/2 cup organic cheese of choice (cheddar, feta, goat cheese, etc)

Optional toppings: avocado, chives, organic cheese

Whisk eggs, veggies, and seasonings in a bowl. In medium pan, heat oil over low-medium heat. Cook 3-4 minutes until mostly cooked, flip the omelet and finish cooking 2-3 minutes. Top with favorite toppings. Can add the cheese in the middle or on top.

Vegetarian Plan Tip: Approved for vegetarians that eat eggs and/or dairy.

Create Your Own Salad

May we suggest putting together a creation of choice. Here are a few ideas...

Mediterranean Style: chicken, cucumbers, feta cheese, red onion, kalamata olives

Simple Salad: meat or fish, any vegetables left over in your fridge, hard-boiled egg

Sweet & Nutty: meat of choice, berries, nuts, gorgonzola or goat cheese

Vegetable Bean Soup
Serves 6 | 60 Minutes

3 tbsp olive or coconut oil
1 small onion, diced
3 carrots, diced
4 stalks of celery, diced
~1/2 cup of parsley (can also
add other spices like sage, if
desired)
2 cloves of garlic, minced
2 cups cabbage (purple or
green)
1 yellow squash, diced
1 zucchini, diced
2 cups kale, chopped
2 cans of cannellini beans,
drained
6 cups of chicken bone
broth or vegetable broth
Salt and pepper to taste
(and garlic powder if you
didn't mince fresh)

Sauté all of the vegetables in oil (except kale and cabbage in large stock pot. Add broth and the rest of the ingredients to the pot and allow to simmer for 30-40 minutes.

DAY 15 | Today's Date _____

Daily Objectives:

- O Watched Daily Teaching
- O Completed 10-Minute Workout + Ab Bonus
- O No Sugar   O 3-6 Servings Healthy Fats & Veggies   O Clean Protein
- O Drank 1/2 My Body Weight In Ounces Of Water
- O Did My Paced Breathing To De-Stress
- O 2 Servings of Detoxing Greens

Challenge Goals:
Write your goals for this 21 Day Challenge below as if you have already accomplished them.

_____

_____

_____

_____

_____

Today, I'm Grateful For:

_____

_____

Health Tracker:

Today I Feel:

☹ ☹ 😐 🙂 😊

− ▭▭▭▭▭▭▭▭ +

I Feel This Way Because:

_____

_____

_____

_____

Almond Butter Blueberry Smoothie

Serves 1 | 10 Minutes

1 large handful of spinach

1/4-1/2 can full-fat coconut milk and/or unsweetened vanilla almond milk

1/2-1 cup frozen blueberries

1 heaping spoonful raw almond butter

1 scoop Livingood Daily Collagen Protein Vanilla

1 tsp Cacao nibs (optional)

1 tsp Flax and/or chia seeds (optional)

Ice (3-4 pieces)

Blend all ingredients in a blender until smooth. Add more milk as needed depending on desired consistency.

Hamburgers

Serves 2 | 30 Minutes

Grill, or cook slowly in coconut oil, hamburger patties with seasoning until preferred temperature. Wrap in romaine lettuce leaves and top with preferred toppings. Cook extra to use as leftover hamburger for lunch or to create a salad the next day.

Vegetarian Plan Tip:
Opt for a black bean burger. Heat the olive oil in a skillet over medium-high heat. Saute the onion until soft, about 5 minutes, then add in the garlic and stir for one more minute. Remove from the heat. In a large bowl, combine the sauteed onion and garlic, beans, sweet potato, ground flax, cumin and salt. Use a fork to stir the mixture, mashing the beans to help the batter stick together. Scoop out the black bean mixture and use your hands to shape it into a burger about 3/4-inch thick. Line a baking sheet with parchment paper. Bake the burgers at 350F for 15 minutes, then use a spatula to gently flip them over and bake for another 5 to 10 minutes.

1 lb grass-fed beef

Salt, pepper, garlic salt (to taste)

Romaine lettuce leaves

Optional Toppings: ketchup, organic cheese, mustard, pickles, onions, avocado, turkey bacon, fried egg, etc

Black Bean Burger (Optional):
2 (15 oz.) cans black beans, drained and rinsed

1 tbsp olive oil

1/2 yellow onion, chopped

3 cloves garlic, minced

1/2 cup mashed sweet potato (steamed, then mashed)

1/4 cup ground flax seeds

1/2 tsp ground cumin

1/2 tsp salt

Cauliflower Tatoes
Serves 2 | 25 Minutes

1 head cauliflower

Salt and pepper, to taste

4 tbsp organic butter

Garlic powder (optional)

Steam cauliflower in steamer until tender. In blender mix cauliflower, butter and seasonings until smooth.

Vegetarian Plan Tip:
Approved for vegetarians that eat eggs and/or dairy.

DAY 16 | Today's Date _____

Daily Objectives:

- O Watched Daily Teaching
- O Completed 10-Minute Workout + Ab Bonus
- O No Sugar   O 3-6 Servings Healthy Fats & Veggies   O Clean Protein
- O Drank 1/2 My Body Weight In Ounces Of Water
- O Did My Paced Breathing To De-Stress
- O 2 Servings of Detoxing Greens

Challenge Goals:
Write your goals for this 21 Day Challenge below as if you have already
accomplished them.

_____

_____

_____

_____

_____

Today, I'm Grateful For:

_____

_____

_____

Health Tracker:

Today I Feel:

☹ ☹ ☺ ☺ ☺
–   +

I Feel This Way Because:

_____

_____

_____

_____

Egg Bites

Yields 6 Muffins | 30 Minutes

8 eggs

1 cup vegetables – diced
(ex: broccoli, bell
peppers, onion,
mushrooms, etc)

1/4 cup almond milk

Salt & pepper (to taste)
(or any other seasoning)

1/2 cup raw or organic
cheese (optional)

1/2 cup turkey bacon,
cooked (optional)

1 tbsp coconut oil

Lightly grease muffin tin with
coconut oil. Whisk all ingredients
together. Pour into muffin tins.
Bake 350 degrees F for 20-25
minutes.

Vegetarian Plan Tip:
Approved for vegetarians that eat
eggs and/or dairy.

You Pick 3

Pick a few of the following items and have a lighter "grazing" lunch! Find your own items to add to your list!

Hard-boiled eggs

Raw veggies & guacamole

Raw veggies & hummus

Turkey & hummus roll ups

Raw organic cheese chunks

Olives

Berries

Apple slices with almond butter

Nuts

Side salad with leftover meat and veggies

Pickles

Smoothie

Chili
Serves 4 | 30 Minutes

1 lb grass fed beef or bison

1 small onion, diced

1 large can organic diced tomatoes

1 small can organic tomato sauce

1-2 cans organic kidney beans

1 can organic black beans (optional)

2 tbsp chili powder

2 tbsp cumin

Salt, pepper, garlic powder (cayenne pepper optional)

Optional toppings: organic sour cream, chives, organic cheese

Brown beef in large pot. Add all other ingredients and simmer until beans are soft. Or can leave all ingredients in a crockpot for a few hours on low. Add toppings as desired.

Vegetarian Plan Tip: Simply remove ground beef/bison and do 2 cans of kidney beans.

DAY 17 | Today's Date _____

Daily Objectives:

- O Watched Daily Teaching
- O Completed 10-Minute Workout + Ab Bonus
- O No Sugar   O 3-6 Servings Healthy Fats & Veggies   O Clean Protein
- O Drank 1/2 My Body Weight In Ounces Of Water
- O Did My Paced Breathing To De-Stress
- O 2 Servings of Detoxing Greens

Challenge Goals:
Write your goals for this 21 Day Challenge below as if you have already accomplished them.

_____

_____

_____

_____

_____

Today, I'm Grateful For:

_____

_____

_____

Health Tracker:

Today I Feel:

☹ ☹ 😐 🙂 😊
– ▢▢▢▢▢▢ +

I Feel This Way Because:

_____

_____

_____

_____

Egg Bites

Yields 6 Muffins | 30 Minutes

8 eggs

1 cup vegetables – diced
(ex: broccoli, bell
peppers, onion,
mushrooms, etc)

1/4 cup almond milk

Salt & pepper (to taste)
(or any other seasoning)

1/2 cup raw or organic
cheese (optional)

1/2 cup turkey bacon,
cooked (optional)

1 tbsp coconut oil

Lightly grease muffin tin with
coconut oil. Whisk all ingredients
together. Pour into muffin tins.
Bake 350 degrees F for 20-25
minutes.

Vegetarian Plan Tip:
Approved for vegetarians that eat
eggs and/or dairy.

Vegetable Stir Fry

Serves 2 | 30 Minutes

Sauté vegetables and seasonings and sauté until tender. Can serve over cauliflower rice if preferred.

4 tbsp coconut oil

Salt, pepper, garlic powder (to taste)

3 tbsp Braggs Liquid Aminos (more or less to taste)

Variety of vegetables: broccoli, bell peppers, onion, snap peas, zucchini, squash, peas, cauliflower, mushrooms, carrots, etc.

NO MORE NUMBNESS & TINGLING, OFF MEDS, NO PAIN, NO MORE HOSPITAL VISITS, ABLE TO WORK!

MORE ENERGY, NO BLOATING, DOWN 10LBS, SLEEPING BETTER, BLOOD PRESSURE LOWERED!

A1C LOWERED, REVERSING DIABATES, AND OFF ALL MEDICATIONS!

NORMAL BP AND CHOLESTEROL AND DOWN 6LBS!

DAY 18 | Today's Date _____

Daily Objectives:

- ○ Watched Daily Teaching
- ○ Completed 10-Minute Workout + Ab Bonus
- ○ No Sugar   ○ 3-6 Servings Healthy Fats & Veggies   ○ Clean Protein
- ○ Drank 1/2 My Body Weight In Ounces Of Water
- ○ Did My Paced Breathing To De-Stress
- ○ 2 Servings of Detoxing Greens

Challenge Goals:
Write your goals for this 21 Day Challenge below as if you have already accomplished them.

_____

_____

_____

_____

_____

Today, I'm Grateful For:

_____

_____

_____

Health Tracker:

Today I Feel:

I Feel This Way Because:

_____

_____

_____

_____

Berry Smoothie

Serves 1 | 10 Minutes

2 handfuls of spinach
and/or kale

1/4-1/2 can of full-fat
coconut milk

1/2 cup of water

1-2 cups of frozen berries
(if using fresh berries add
3-4 ice cubes)

1 scoop Livingood Daily
Collagen Protein Vanilla

Combine all ingredients in a
high-powered blender and mix.
Use more or less of any ingredient
to make thicker, thinner, or colder.

Cesar Salad

Serves 2 | 20 Minutes

Mix or blend all dressing ingredients together until smooth. Combine chicken, spinach, romaine, and dressing in a bowl with a lid and shake until completely covered. Add more parmesan cheese to the top before eating.

Vegetarian Plan Tip:
Simply remove cooked chicken.

2 chicken breasts, cooked how desired

Organic spinach and romaine lettuce

Dressing:
1/2 cup olive oil

1 lemon (juiced, can add zest as well)

1/3 cup parmesan cheese

4 tsp dijon mustard (no sugar)

1-2 garlic cloves or garlic powder

Worcestershire sauce, to taste (no sugar)

Salt and pepper, to taste

Steak Fajitas
Serves 2 | 45 Minutes

2 tbsp coconut oil

1 medium sized steak of choice

1 small red onion

2 organic red bell peppers

1 organic green bell pepper

Spinach or romaine lettuce

Seasoning: 2 tbsp chili powder, 3 tbsp cumin, salt, pepper, garlic powder

Optional Toppings: raw organic cheddar cheese, black beans, organic sour cream, cilantro, cucumber, avocado, salsa

Saute steak in coconut oil over medium heat until cooked. Add vegetables and seasoning (may add a little water to help steam the vegetables) Cook until vegetables are tender. Put on a plate of spinach and top with desired toppings.

DAY 19 | Today's Date _____

Daily Objectives:

O Watched Daily Teaching

O Completed 10-Minute Workout + Ab Bonus

O No Sugar   O 3-6 Servings Healthy Fats & Veggies   O Clean Protein

O Drank 1/2 My Body Weight In Ounces Of Water

O Did My Paced Breathing To De-Stress

O 2 Servings of Detoxing Greens

Challenge Goals:
Write your goals for this 21 Day Challenge below as if you have already
accomplished them.

_____

_____

_____

_____

_____

Today, I'm Grateful For:

_____

_____

_____

Health Tracker:

Today I Feel:

– ⊏━━━━━━━⊐ +

I Feel This Way Because:

_____

_____

_____

_____

Egg Scramble

Serves 1 | 20 Minutes

2 eggs

1/2 cup vegetables (bell peppers, spinach, zucchini, mushrooms, broccoli, onion, etc)

1/2 cup turkey bacon or turkey sausage, cooked (optional)

Salt, pepper (to taste)

2 tbsp coconut oil

Optional toppings: avocado, cheese, (cheddar, feta, goat, etc), chives

Whisk eggs, veggies, pre-cooked meat, and seasonings in a bowl. In a medium pan, heat oil over medium-low heat. Cook 6-8 minutes until eggs are cooked through. Top with favorite toppings.

Vegetarian Plan Tip: Approved for vegetarians that eat eggs and/or dairy. Avoid turkey bacon/sausage and sautee another 1/2 cup of veggies of your choice if desired.

Meatloaf

Serves 4 | 60 Minutes

Mix all ingredients well in a bowl. Transfer to a lightly coconut oil greased loaf pan, pack lightly. Bake 1 hour or until cooked through at 350 degrees F. Can top with a little ketchup if desired. Can serve with Mashed Cauliflower Tatoes recipe.

1 1/2 pounds grass-fed ground beef

1 egg

1 small onion, diced

1/2 cup organic ketchup (no sugar) (can use tomato paste also)

2 tbsp Braggs Liquid Amino Acids

2 tsp organic Worcestershire sauce

Salt, pepper, garlic powder, to taste

Optional: healthy cracker (such as Simple Mills, Mary's Gone Crackers or Akmak crackers, finely crushed)

Cauliflower Tatoes

Serves 2 | 25 Minutes

1 head cauliflower

Salt and pepper, to taste

4 tbsp organic butter

Garlic powder (optional)

Steam cauliflower in steamer until tender. In blender mix cauliflower, butter and seasonings until smooth.

Vegetarian Plan Tip: Approved for vegetarians that eat eggs and/or dairy.

DAY 20 | Today's Date _____

Daily Objectives:

- O Watched Daily Teaching
- O Completed 10-Minute Workout + Ab Bonus
- O No Sugar   O 3-6 Servings Healthy Fats & Veggies   O Clean Protein
- O Drank 1/2 My Body Weight In Ounces Of Water
- O Did My Paced Breathing To De-Stress
- O 2 Servings of Detoxing Greens

Challenge Goals:
Write your goals for this 21 Day Challenge below as if you have already accomplished them.

_____

_____

_____

_____

_____

Today, I'm Grateful For:

_____

_____

_____

Health Tracker:

Today I Feel:

☹ 🙁 😐 🙂 😀
− [============] +

I Feel This Way Because:

_____

_____

_____

_____

Smoothie Bowl

Serves 1 | 15 Minutes

1/2-1 cup coconut or
almond milk

1 1/2 cup frozen berries of
choice (acai,
blueberries, blackberries,
strawberries, raspberries,
etc. - can add 1/2 fresh or
frozen banana for thicker
consistency)

1/2 scoop Livingood Daily
Collagen Protein Vanilla
(optional)

Ice to thicken
consistency, if desired

Optional Toppings: sliced
fruit or berries, coconut
flakes, chia seeds, cacao
nibs or 70% or greater
stevia sweetened dark
chocolate chips

Put all ingredients in a
high-powered blender or food
processor and blend until thick,
smoothie-like consistency. Add more ice
or berries if you prefer thicker bowls.
Pour the smoothie bowl mixture into a
bowl and top with your favorite
toppings! Enjoy immediately!

Turkey Bacon Cheeseburger Casserole
Serves 6 | 60 Minutes

Make cauliflower mashed tatoes and set aside. Cook turkey bacon in large skillet and set aside, keep the bacon grease in pan. Add ground beef to the same skillet and cook until browned. Add the seasonings and set aside. For the sauce: add butter in a pan and stir in the flour over low heat (can use the same pan as hamburger if you want more flavor). Cook until the flour has absorbed the butter and then add heavy cream and mustard. Cook until the sauce thickens. In a 9×13 baking dish place half of the sauce on the bottom of the dish. Spread the cauliflower tatoes as evenly as possible in the dish. Sprinkle half of the bag of cheese over the tatoes. Sprinkle on the ground beef. Pour the other half of the sauce over the beef. Sprinkle remaining cheddar cheese over the sauce and sprinkle the top with the bacon. Cover and bake on 350 degrees F for approximately 30 minutes. Allow to cool a bit before serving.

1 package of Turkey Bacon, cooked and cut into bite-sized pieces

1 1/2 lb Grass Fed Beef

1 head Cauliflower, cooked and made into mashed cauliflower tatoes

Salt, Pepper, Garlic Powder, Onion Powder (optional)

Sauce:
3 tbsp yellow mustard
2 tbsp Butter

1 1/2 cup organic heavy cream

1/3 cup coconut flour

1 (8 ounce) package organic cheddar cheese

LOST 4 BELT NOTCHES DURING THE 21 DAY CHALLENGE!

BETTY IS OFF OF 9 OUT OF 11 MEDICATIONS AND HER CARPAL TUNNEL IS GONE!

27 YEARS OF NUMBNESS/TINGLING, HIGH BLOOD PRESSURE & DIABETES GONE!

DAY 21 | Today's Date _____

Daily Objectives:

- O Watched Daily Teaching
- O Completed 10-Minute Workout + Ab Bonus
- O No Sugar   O 3-6 Servings Healthy Fats & Veggies   O Clean Protein
- O Drank 1/2 My Body Weight In Ounces Of Water
- O Did My Paced Breathing To De-Stress
- O 2 Servings of Detoxing Greens

Challenge Goals:
Write your goals for this 21 Day Challenge below as if you have already accomplished them.

_____

_____

_____

_____

_____

Today, I'm Grateful For:

_____

_____

_____

Health Tracker:

Today I Feel:

– [☹ ☹ 😐 🙂 😀] +

I Feel This Way Because:

_____

_____

_____

_____

Vegetable Omelet
Serves 1 | 15 Minutes

3 eggs

1 cup vegetables (bell peppers, spinach, onion, broccoli, mushrooms, asparagus, etc)

Salt, pepper (to taste)

2 tbsp coconut oil

1/2 cup organic cheese of choice (cheddar, feta, goat cheese, etc)

Optional toppings: avocado, chives, organic cheese

Whisk eggs, veggies, and seasonings in a bowl. In medium pan, heat oil over low-medium heat. Cook 3-4 minutes until mostly cooked, flip the omelet and finish cooking 2-3 minutes. Top with favorite toppings. Can add the cheese in the middle or on top.

Vegetarian Plan Tip: Approved for vegetarians that eat eggs and/or dairy.

Grill Fish or Meat & Vegetable of Choice
Serves 2 | 30 Minutes

Pretty simple here! Grill and season your chicken as desired. Season as desired or add a little organic butter on top! Prepare your vegetables as desired, cube and saute, bake, grill, etc.

2 organic chicken breasts

Salt, pepper, garlic powder (to taste)

1 vegetable of choice (squash, zucchini, broccoli, brussels sprouts, etc)

CONGRATULATIONS

Congratulations! You have started a habit of building real health. However, health is a journey, not a destination, and you're just getting started! Keep the course, continue to build health, and take care of your biggest asset... you!

Don't leave others behind! Now that you know what you know, help someone. 99% of people have never experienced real health the way you just have. There are thousands of people within a ten-mile radius of you right now praying and pleading for an answer to their health problems. If they keep waiting for and managing sickness and disease they will keep having sickness and disease. If they build health they'll get health. Their answer may just be in your seat.

YOU ARE THE SOLUTION!

You could save their life just by inviting them to the challenge and it doesn't cost you a thing to do it. So your last challenge today is, who is one person you will share this information with? Will you be the solution for real health care?

LET'S CELEBRATE

LIFE CHANGE IS WORTH CELEBRATING!

Enter to win and vote for the Challenge Champion!

TO ENTER TO WIN THE $500 GRAND PRIZE:

In the Facebook group, film and post a 60 second or less video and include your written testimonial answering the following 3 questions:

1. What were your problems before the challenge?
   (ex. pain, weight, meds, disease, conditions, etc.)
2. What results have you seen throughout the challenge?
   (ex. weight loss, energy, off medications, lower blood pressure, improved blood work, etc.)
3. What would you say to someone thinking about doing the challenge?

TO VOTE FOR THE CHALLENGE CHAMPION:

Voting will be live in your Livingood Daily Challenge Facebook group during the final week.

ANNOUNCING THE CHALLENGE CHAMPION:

The winner of Challenge Champion will be announced in your Livingood Daily Challenge Facebook group during the final week!

NEXT STEPS

Congratulations on finishing your Livingood Daily Challenge! This was your Quickstart on your journey to experience real health. It's a journey because we never arrive; there is always a next step for all of us when it comes to health. If you stop your new healthy habits what happens? You go back to where you came from and no one wants that. Have you hit your ultimate health goal yet? Chances are no but you are now ready to go further on this journey and get more advanced. Because of that, we have 2 simple next steps for you:

Ready to turn this into a Lifestyle?

1 If you love having access to the 10-Minute Workouts, Recipes, and Real Health Solutions, you have the opportunity to be a part of the Livingood Daily Lifestyle. You'll get ongoing Challenges and access to the workouts, trainings, and health guides. Visit livingooddaily.com to learn more.

2 Still dealing with a certain condition? Customize your next Challenge with our condition specific bundles to get the natural remedies and specific guides to use during your next Livingood Daily Challenge. Visit livingooddaily.com to learn more.

THE LIVINGOOD DAILY LIFESTYLE